Mary's

CANNABIS PRIMERS
COLLECTION

VOLUME I

This volume includes:
Issue #1 Introduction to Cannabis Science
Issue #2 Cannabis and Cancer
Issue #3 The Endocannabinoid System
Issue #4 Cannabis & Nutrition

Edited by: Alice O'Leary Randall

Editor-in-Chief: Alice O'Leary Randall
Design: Jesica Clark
Contributors: Patrick Allen, Jessica Aragona, Joseph Cohen, D.O., Bonni S.
Goldstein, M.D., Heather Jackson, Justin Kander, Noel Palmer, Ph.D., Marla
Perez, Graham Sorkin, and Dustin Sulak, D.O..
Special Thanks to: Cannabis.info, Cannabis Now, Leafly.com, and NORML.

Published by: Mary's Medicinals

This publication was produced by Mary's Medicinals and Mary's Nutritionals in consultation with medical professionals and scientists. However, our understanding of cannabis medicine is constantly evolving and so we can only share what we have learned from patients and the research that is currently available. Every patient will have individual reactions to different treatments Use of this information is not intended to be a substitute for professional medical judgment and you should promptly contact your own health care provider regarding any medical conditions or medical questions that you have or before beginning any treatment.

Mary's Cannabis Primer is published as an educational resource about the benefits of cannabis. It is part of Mary's commitment to educating the general public about this remarkable plant. For further information please visit: www.maryspubs.com.

ISBN: 978-0692096161

Mary's Medicinals • Denver, CO • MarysMedicinals.com
www.MarysPubs.com

TABLE OF CONTENTS

About this Book 1

Issue #1: Introduction to Cannabis Science 2

Introduction to Cannabis Science 4

CBD - The Basics 6

Mary's Medicinals Selection Chart 8

How Did We Get Here? 10

Issue #2: Cannabis and Cancer 19

Cannabis & Cancer 22

Cannabis Use for Pediatric Cancers 25

Bobby & His Kids: Portrait of an Activist 28

Jonah's Story 30

The Bud Tender is NOT a Doctor 32

Industry Collaboration Helps to Educate and Empower
Patients Interested in Exploring Cannabinoid Therapy 34

What is Cannabis Oil? 35

Legally Available Cannabis-Like Medicines 36

Cannabis Man 38

Issue #3: The Endocannabinoid System 41

Chronic Pain & Medical Cannabis 44

The Endocannabinoid System: A Physician's Perspective 47

Medical Cannabis Laws Map 52

Here's the Thing: A Mother's Story 55

How to Find It: Searching for Medical Cannabis
Information 57

Issue #4: Cannabis & Nutrition 61

The Incredibly Versatile Cannabis Plant 63

A Dietician's Perspective on Cannabis 65

Nutrition and Cannabis 67

Healthy! Nutritional Value of Hemp Seeds 69

Cannabis and a Healthy Lifestyle 71

Sam Skipper and the Nutritional Power of Cannabis 73

Hemp or Cannabis? Which is More Nutritional? 74

Glossary 76

ABOUT THIS BOOK

In 2015 the first issue of *Mary's Cannabis Primer* was published. The idea was simple: pick a facet of the medical cannabis issue and focus on explaining it in detail. The goal was to provide the "prime information" needed by an educated medical cannabis patient or caregiver, many of whom are coming to the cannabis issue for the first time.

Yet even the most seasoned cannabis researcher is apt to admit deficiencies in their knowledge because the knowledge base is expanding so rapidly. The one thing we can say with some certainty is that we have only scratched the surface of cannabis' therapeutic and health potential. This fact makes the concept of *The Primer* even more important. There is a constant need to re-evaluate previous knowledge and place it in context with current discovery.

The Primers seemed to strike a chord with the public and it was not uncommon for Mary's Medicinals to re-print various issues because of demand. At a certain point that becomes impractical so Mary's adopted the strategy of providing single issues via the Mary's Publications website page (www. maryspubs.com) and for those who want printed copy this Collection, available via amazon.com, fills the bill.

Mary's was founded in 2013 and in the five years of operation the company has grown and evolved with new products and new looks. But the fundamentals remain the same, providing the best product available and educating the public about this remarkable plant. On behalf of Mary's Medicinals and Mary's Nutritionals, thank you for supporting our efforts to educate the public with regard to the medical, health and nutritional value of cannabis. We hope you enjoy this Collection.

Alice O'Leary Randall
Editor-in-Chief, *Mary's Cannabis Primer*

Mary's

CANNABIS PRIMER

issue #1

INTRODUCTION TO CANNABIS SCIENCE

CBD - The Basics
Mary's Medicinals Selection Guide
How Did We Get Here?

EDITOR'S NOTE

Welcome to the first issue of *Mary's Cannabis Primer*, published by Mary's Foundation for Caring and made available to dispensaries and organizations free-of-charge. Our goal is simple: to provide an ongoing source of educational information about the medical uses of cannabis.

There are dozens of medical cannabis publications available and literally thousands of websites. It is an exciting and dynamic time in the history of medical cannabis. Research is expanding rapidly and politically there is a new awareness of the plant's value and the need for legislative reform. Also exciting is the expanding knowledge with respect to the chemistry of cannabis and the new methods of cultivation that are yielding even more opportunities for therapeutic application. Often lost in the shuffle are the basic facts about cannabis as well as the history. *Mary's Cannabis Primer* will focus on these basic building blocks–history and research–to bring to our readers a better understanding of the fundamentals of this important public health issue.

Our first issue is dedicated to the beginnings of the medical cannabis issue as well as some basic chemistry and terms that are helpful in understanding cannabis. Because cannabis is a plant and not a synthetically produced drug, it becomes important for the patients (i.e., the consumer) to understand as much as possible about how the plants are developed and what makes one plant different from another. This can be a daunting task but the rewards are many. Our hope is that *Mary's Cannabis Primer* will help patients and their caregivers to better understand this miraculous plant.

Alice O'Leary-Randall
Executive Editor - Mary's Cannabis Primer

INTRODUCTION TO CANNABIS SCIENCE

Dr. Noel Palmer is chief scientist at Mary's Medicinals. Recently *Mary's Cannabis Primer* executive editor Alice O'Leary-Randall talked to Noel about the cannabis plant.

Noel, there was a time when using cannabis medically consisted of using whatever the dealer had to offer but in today's world there is a vast array of choices and an enormous amount of information. I'm hoping you can help our readers sort out some of this chemistry stuff. Let's start at the beginning. What is cannabis?

Cannabis is a plant that produces many phytochemicals, which simply means chemical compounds that occur naturally in plants. Most interesting to humans are the cannabinoids, a phytochemical that research has shown stimulates the endocannabinoid system – the chemical receptor system that has been found in all mammals, including, of course, humans. Cannabis is an annual flowering plant, with distinct male and female plants (which makes it dioecious). It is most closely related to hops. Historically, cannabis has been used for fiber, oils from pressed seeds, therapeutic applications and as a recreational drug.

Are these naturally occurring cannabinoids the chemicals that produce the therapeutic effect?

Yes and no. Naturally occurring cannabinoids are acidic. If you look at the chemical structure of a natural cannabinoid you'll see that it has an extra group on the molecular backbone of the ingredient. In its natural state (diagram 1) cannabinoid is acidic and these acidic cannabinoids are not active in the human body the same way that neutral cannabinoids are. The endocannabinoid system looks for neutral cannabinoids and naturally occurring cannabinoids become neutral through a process called "decarboxylation."

Sounds really complicated. How does this "decarboxylation" happen?

People have been, in many cases, unknowingly activating these acidic cannabinoids by smoking or baking with cannabis – two processes that use heat/energy. Typically, this energy is sufficient to decarboxylate and/or vaporize the cannabinoids. The energy (from light or heat) causes the carboxylic acid functional group to fall off the molecular structure and we get "neutral" cannabinoids – such as delta-9 THC, which bind to the endocannabinoid receptors and provide a therapeutic effect.

But some people claim that ingesting raw cannabis is therapeutic too.

Recent research has shown that the acidic cannabinoids may have therapeutic potential apart from the neutral cannabinoids, showing efficacy in stimulating the auto-immune system in humans. Many people are now juicing cannabis as a result. Research with raw cannabis is truly in its infancy. The focus has been on decarboxylated (i.e. smoked) cannabis because that has been the primary method of using the plant for the past 50-75 years but there is historical evidence of cultures consuming raw cannabis, literally "grazing" from the plant.

Many people are confused about the "types" of cannabis. Can you talk about this?

While cannabis lies in a single genus or category, there are many sub-species (or species) that are described by cannabis users and cultivators. Probably the best known examples of these classifications are indica and sativa.

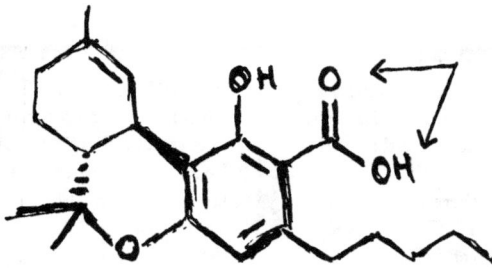

(DIAGRAM 1)

Generally cannabis plants can be broken into two major types, the fiber-type and the drug-type. The fiber-type of cannabis grows very tall with minimal flower formation and is known as hemp. Returning once again to our phytochemicals, the fiber-type of cannabis will generally express CBDA as a primary cannabinoid.

The therapeutic or recreational type of cannabis generally grows with more defined flowers and, depending on the location and species (indica, sativa, ruderalus), it will grow tall or shorter. This type cannabis generally expresses an abundance of the phytochemical THCA which is the acidic form of the neutralized THC.

So, does that mean CBD is a neutralized form of CBDA?
Exactly! CBDA is predominant in the fiber-form of cannabis, better known as hemp. Modern breeding work by cultivars has been able to take some of this CBDA and breed it into

a drug-type cannabis. This has created "mutants" that grow like the drug-type cannabis but mainly express CBDA. These mutants are generally shorter with very clear flowers and lots of trichomes.

What are trichomes?
Trichomes are very small, appendages on the flower of the cannabis plants that are the production factories and storage locations for all cannabinoids and terpenes. Trichomes give cannabis the "frosty" appearance– sometimes making the plant white/silver on the surface. There are a few different types of trichomes, but most prevalent in cannabis are the glandular trichomes which produce and store cannabinoids and terpenes. There is a common mis-conception that cannabis produces cannabinoids that are imbedded in the plant material. In fact, all cannabinoids are on the surface of the plant in these trichomes. Some have speculated that the presence of these trichomes on the surface of the plant has been a

natural evolution of the plant to guard itself from the sun's powerful UV radiation and/or plant infestation.

So would these trichomes contain the medical CBD, like Charlotte's Web™, that we hear about so much?
CBD is CBD regardless of source (hemp vs drug types). Many people think that hemp derived CBD is not as valid as CBD derived from a "drug-type" cannabis. Same with THC but that is not the case. Many people believe that the subtle differences in cannabis are not with the cannabinoids, but rather the terpenes.

And how do terpenes differ from trichomes?
Modern research on cannabis biochemistry has suggested that terpenes are in fact intimately involved in the production of cannabinoids – serving as starting compounds in the biosynthetic pathway. These biochemical reactions occur in the trichomes of the plant. ✹

CBD - THE BASICS

CBD has been getting a lot of press attention because of its reported ability to stop seizures in pediatric epilepsy patients. Additionally, there are numerous online sites, including Mary's Nutritionals Elite CBD, that offer nutritional products made from "legal" CBD. So, what's the difference between CBD from cannabis and CBD from hemp?

From a legal and scientific perspective, there are two varieties of the Cannabis plant. Cannabis which contains more than 0.3% THC (the component that causes psychoactive effects – "getting high") and is sometimes called drug-type cannabis. The other is hemp cannabis – which contains less than 0.3% THC, and does not cause any psychoactive effects. It is legal for farmers to grow and is sometimes called fiber-type cannabis. Businesses craft clothing, soaps, nutritional products and even cars and houses out of hemp cannabis. Hemp cannabis is legal across the United States and most of the world. Both types of cannabis contain cannabidiol (CBD) molecules. It is interesting to note that plants other than cannabis and hemp contain CBD. These include flax and azaleas.

So is there a difference between CBD derived from hemp and CBD derived from cannabis or flax? Nope, the CBD molecule itself is the same, regardless of from which plant it is extracted. However, many hemp CBD products are imported from places like China where plants are grown with pesticides and exposed to heavy metals and pollution. When processed, this hemp extract contains toxins and heavy metals. The Food and Drug Administration (FDA) has reported that some of these imported extracts don't even contain any active CBD. Last year, the Drug Enforcement Administration (DEA) stated that, "Because it is illicitly produced by clandestine manufacturers, its actual content is uncertain and will vary depending on the source of the material."

To provide an alternative to these potentially dangerous foreign sources, American companies including Mary's Nutritionals have begun to work directly with farms, including several in Colorado, to cultivate high-CBD hemp plants. One of these farms is Elite Botanicals - a family-run organic hemp farm that produces Elite CBD plants in full compliance with Colorado Department of Agriculture, the 2014 Farm Bill and the pending Industrial Hemp Farming Act of 2015. The Elite CBD™ extracted from these plants is distributed nationwide.

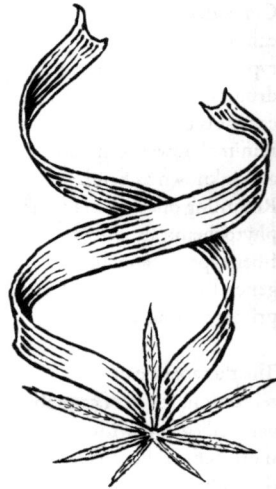

"We've seen firsthand the potential of the cannabis plant to change people's lives," said Nicole Smith, founder & CEO, Mary's Nutritionals & Mary's Medicinals. "The FDA prevents us from educating the public about cannabinoids, however, the federal government holds a patent on CBD which clearly states some of the benefits that patients across the country, and especially in Colorado, are reporting." The United States Department of Health and Human Services holds patent 6,630,507, which states that: "Cannabidiol has been studied as an antiepileptic. Cannabinoids have been found to have antioxidant properties ... useful in the treatment of wide variety of oxidation associated diseases, inflammatory and autoimmune diseases. Cannabinoids are found to have particular application as neuroprotectants, for example in limiting neurological damage following ischemic insults, such as stroke and trauma, or in the treatment of neurodegenerative diseases, such as Alzheimer's disease, Parkinson's disease and HIV dementia."

"With so many people travelling to Colorado to access CBD, we felt that it was our responsibility to make quality, domestically grown CBD available to everyone who seeks it for any reason," said Smith.

PATIENT STORY: CBD FOR PTSD

During a walking patrol in Kandahar, Afghanistan, US Army Veteran Matt D. was severely injured by an improvised explosive device. He now suffers from PTSD, traumatic brain injury, insomnia, debilitating migraines and chronic pain.

He was awarded a Purple Heart for his valor. Matt was treated by the Veterans Administration with

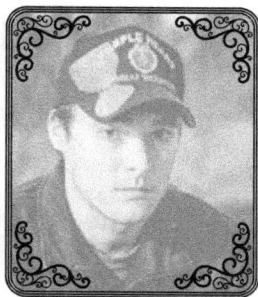

U.S. Army veteran, Matt D.

dozens of prescription drugs including OxyContin and codeine in an attempt to control his pain and allow him to sleep.

Matt began using cannabis to relieve his pain and promote sleep. He uses CBD patches for his migraines, and CBN patches to sleep. Like many patients, he uses a CBD transdermal gel pen to stop migraines quickly as they start.

Support Veterans through groups such as:

• Operation Grow4Vets
• Veterans for Compassionate Care
• Enigami Veterans Post Traumatic Stress & Medical Cannabis Study
• Wounded Warrior Project

TRACK YOUR MEDS WITH MARY'S JOURNAL!

Research on medical cannabis is expanding rapidly but there is still a lack of good, patient-oriented data. This type of data is one component of evidence-based practice (EBP) which

is particularly well suited for medical cannabis since so much of the data is contingent on the physician-patient relationship. Sharing information will help many patients in the coming years as we work together to advance understanding and use of canna-based medicine.

Mary's Journal is a mobile app that helps patients monitor and optimize their cannabis healthcare, while gathering anonymous data on use preferences, patterns and results. This data increases the body of knowledge available to researchers and patients, and in turn promotes better use of cannabis medicine and the creation of better products.

Patients that use Mary's Journal join a unique community focused on sharing information to improve canna-based medicine for patients around the world. Mary's Journal is your opportunity to be a part of medical history.

Look for Mary's Journal in the App Store and Google Play Store. ✳

Mary's

MEDICINALS

SELECTION GUIDE

CAN•NAB•I•NOID

/'kanəbəˌnoid,kə'nabə-/

Cannabinoids are the chemical compounds within cannabis that are reported to relieve a variety of ailments. Cannabinoids replicate endocannabinoids, compounds our bodies naturally produce to balance and control communication between cells. Researchers believe that unpleasant symptoms and diseases occur when a deficiency or problem affects the endocannabinoid system.

PATCHES

	CBD	CBD: THC	CBN	THCa	THC INDICA
ANALGESIC	✓	✓	✓	✓	✓
ANTI-ARTHRITIC		✓	✓	✓	✓
ANTI-BACTERIAL	✓	✓			
ANTI-CONVULSIVE	✓	✓	✓	✓	✓
ANTI-EMETIC	✓	✓	✓	✓	✓
ANTI-EPILEPTIC	✓	✓	✓	✓	✓
ANTI-PROLIFERATIVE	✓			✓	✓
ANTI-INFLAMMATORY	✓	✓	✓	✓	✓
ANTI-SPASMODIC	✓	✓	✓	✓	✓
APPETITE STIMULANT					✓
BLOOD SUGAR BALANCING	✓				
ENERGY SUPPORT				✓	
GASTROINTESTINAL RELIEF	✓	✓	✓	✓	✓
IMMUNE SUPPORT	✓	✓	✓	✓	
NEUROPROTECTIVE	✓			✓	
NON-PSYCHOACTIVE	✓	✓	✓	✓	
SLEEP SUPPORT	✓	✓	✓	✓	✓
STRESS / ANXIETY RELIEF	✓	✓	✓	✓	✓

TRANSDERMAL PATCHES: With a quick onset and unsurpassed duration, Mary's award-winning patches are easy to adhere discreetly to any part of the skin for up to 12 hours of relief.

TRANSDERMAL GELS: A perfect resource for managing breakthrough pain or creating blended cannabinoid ratios, Mary's gel pens offer rapid onset and duration of 4-6 hours.

CAPSULES: Designed for patients that need a long lasting, slow release dose of cannabinoids for regular use.

COMPOUND: Applied topically, Mary's compound is reported to help with pain, inflammation and muscle soreness with nearly immediate onset, and duration of 2-4 hours.

GELS					CAPSULES		COMPOUND	
THC SATIVA	CBD	CBN	THC INDICA	THC SATIVA	CBD	CBN	CBC	CBD: THC
	✓	✓	✓		✓	✓	✓	✓
✓	✓	✓	✓	✓	✓	✓	✓	✓
	✓				✓		✓	
✓	✓	✓	✓	✓	✓	✓		
✓	✓	✓	✓	✓	✓	✓		
✓	✓	✓	✓	✓	✓	✓		
✓	✓		✓	✓	✓		✓	✓
✓	✓	✓	✓	✓	✓	✓	✓	✓
✓	✓	✓	✓	✓	✓	✓	✓	✓
✓			✓	✓	✓			
	✓				✓			
✓				✓				
	✓	✓	✓		✓	✓	✓	✓
	✓	✓			✓	✓		
	✓				✓			
	✓	✓			✓	✓	✓	✓
	✓	✓	✓		✓	✓		
✓	✓	✓	✓	✓	✓	✓		

2018 Version

HOW DID WE GET HERE?

By Alice O'Leary-Randall

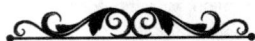

A true medical cannabis pioneer, Alice has worked for nearly four decades to expand medical access to cannabis. She is the widow of America's first legal medical marijuana patient, Robert C. Randall. She is executive editor of *Mary's Cannabis Primer*, serves on the Board of Directors for Mary's Foundation for Caring and American Cannabis Nurses Association.

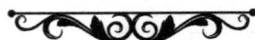

There was a time in the not so distant past when using medical cannabis was a relatively straightforward process. From the 1970s to the early 2000s, medical use of marijuana basically took one form—smoked. If you needed the drug medically you found a dealer, secured the product and rolled a joint. You smoked until your symptoms disappeared. Potency was erratic, as was supply. It was not something you discussed with your healthcare providers and if they expressed wonderment and confusion at the improvement of your condition you held your tongue and smiled quietly.

Today all of that has changed. Almost one-half of the states have laws authorizing the medical use of cannabis. A score of states have the so-called CBD-only laws that allow legal access to one of the components of cannabis. Even in states that have not yet legalized medical cannabis there are legal, non-psychoactive alternatives—made from hemp, the first cousin of cannabis—that can provide significant therapeutic effect to individuals with a wide variety of ailments.

In states with legalized access there is often a dizzying array of choices for the medical patient: cannabis buds labeled with exotic names such as OMG Kush and Purple Haze, pre-rolled cannabis cigarettes, tinctures, edibles, salves, creams, pills, suppositories and transdermal patches. How did we get here? To answer that question some background is required.

A BRIEF HISTORY

At the turn of the 20th Century cannabis was widely used for a variety of ailments. More than 2,000 preparations of the plant were available and the preparations were prescribed for a wide variety of ailments. The Marijuana Tax Act of 1937, enacted for racial and economic

purposes, began the demise of medical cannabis use but it was hastened by the advent of many new pharmaceutical drugs such as penicillin and digitalis, each derived from natural products but suddenly available in "pure" and "modern" dosing. Cannabis might have survived this dawning of the new age of pharmaceuticals but the U.S. federal government – using a slang term for the plant — had branded marijuana a "dangerous drug" and was engaged in a systematic destruction of the plant's long and distinguished use as a medication. The drug was removed from the *U.S. Pharmacopeia* in 1942.

Medical use of cannabis never fully disappeared but it was relegated to the category of "folk medicine" which, in the 1940s and 50s, had a disparaging connotation. And obtaining the plant became more and more difficult.

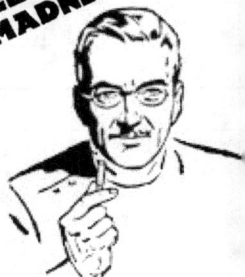

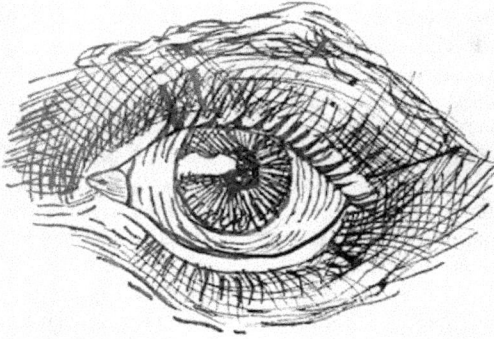

Glaucoma is a disease caused by elevated pressure within the eyeball.

In the 1960s and 70s there was a reawakening of interest in the medical use of cannabis. This was generated by "anecdotal" reports from marijuana users but also from researchers of the federal government who were charged with finding the "harms" of marijuana but very often stumbled upon potential benefits. Some researchers reported these benefits publicly. Glaucoma is a good example. Researchers were seeking a way to detect illegal marijuana use and a popular myth had been that smoking marijuana causes bloodshot eyes. That theory was debunked but researchers did note that smoking marijuana caused a lowering of inner eye pressure and Dr. Robert Hepler of UCLA wrote a letter to the *Journal of the American Medical Association* (JAMA) in September, 1971 stating that:

The purpose of this letter is to present preliminary data concerning the most impressive change observed thus far, namely a substantial decrease in the intraocular pressure observed in a large percentage of subject....The possible implications, including the mechanism of action, and even possible therapeutic action in the treatment of glaucoma, are obvious.

BIRTH OF A MOVEMENT

Five years later a 28-year old college professor in Washington, D.C made medical and legal history when he proved in criminal and civil law proceedings that marijuana was a "medical necessity." Randall was tested at UCLA, by Dr. Hepler, for ten days. The results were incontrovertible: without the addition of marijuana conventional medications were ineffective for Randall. Armed with this data, the young man successfully petitioned the federal government for access to U.S. supplies of marijuana and became "America's Only Legal Pot Smoker." Robert C. Randall would lead the fight for medical access to cannabis for the next 25 years and is the acknowledged father of the medical marijuana movement.

But even Randall's legal access demonstrates the rudimentary state of cannabis research as well as the intense level of prohibition in the later part of the 20th Century. There was one source for medical marijuana, the federal government, and the product was grown solely with a view towards the psychoactive properties of the plant. Even though numerous constituents of the plant were already known, it was only delta-9 THC, the ingredient that gets people "high," that interested the government. The plant was grown in Mississippi and then shipped to North Carolina where it was processed and rolled into cigarettes. The government claimed that all other ingredients were "removed" at this point and the cigarettes were purely delta-9 THC, dose-quantified in the 1.5 to 1.8% range. The government also created a delta-9 THC pill that delivered 10mg of THC. The pill was not intended for human consumption but did facilitate animal experiments.

CANNABIS AND THE ECS

In the early 1990s a series of research discoveries led to discovery of the endocannabinoid system (ECS). At about the same time the legal situation in the U.S. changed dramatically as medical cannabis patients began employing the ballot initiative process to legalize medical cannabis. The first was in 1996 in California. Not surprisingly the Californians embraced medical cannabis wholeheartedly and the loose structure of Proposition 215 allowed a free-wheeling industry and unregulated market to develop in the Gold Rush state. California's state program remains one of the least restrictive in the country. It is also not surprising that the early years of the program drew upon the thriving, albeit still illegal, recreational market for product supplies and marketing.

Thus cannabis medications took on a decidedly non-medical veneer. Patients ordered medicines by their street names—e.g. OG Kush and Purple Urkle—and "medical dispensaries" looked much more like "head shops" than pharmacies. For the marijuana-naïve patient it was a foreign and frightening world.

As we entered the 21st Century, however, things began to change...somewhat. Clinical research outside of the U.S. began looking at the various cannabinoids, especially the now-famous CBD, and their effect on the ECS. As it became clear that the ECS was a pivotal component of human biology and is a key player in the important process of homeostasis, the research accelerated. New applications of the cannabis plant emerged, fulfilling the prescient testimony of the AMA lobbyist Dr. William Woodward who, in 1937, spoke against the Marijuana Tax. Acknowledging that the plant was falling into disuse he also wisely noted that "future investigation may show that there are substantial medical uses for Cannabis."

The good doctor would be amazed. As it became clear that cannabis has a critical effect on homeostasis, the intellectual curiosity of researchers around the globe was piqued. For researchers, cannabis was suddenly an exciting "new drug" and many began to explore therapeutic application possibilities heretofore unthought-of with respect to cannabis— diabetes, Alzheimer's disease, Parkinson's, ALS, anti-tumor properties, and control of some pesky new "super-bugs" such as MRSA and even Ebola. Concurrent with the explosion in intellectual curiosity there was a blossoming of American entrepreneur spirit in those states that had legalized cannabis. Unshackled by federal government regulation, cannabis growers in states such as Colorado and California began exploring the plant and delivery systems. Whatever your interest might be— horticulture, chemistry, culinary delights, mechanical delivery devices, marketing, business development— the new cannabis growth industry had a place for you. The Green Rush was on and the result would be a boon for those using cannabis medically.

PRESENT DAY

In the late 1990s, with just a handful of states authorizing medical cannabis, energies of the cannabis industry entrepreneurs were focused primarily on the very "newness" of their situation as they carefully maneuvered through a minefield of federal, state and local regulations. For at least five years after passage of Proposition 215 raids by the Drug Enforcement Administration (DEA) were fairly common place in California. Very often the purpose seemed to be disruption and intimidation rather than actual arrests. If the purpose of these raids was "to keep the lid on" and discourage other states from passing medical cannabis laws then the tactic failed. One-by-one other states followed the electoral lead of California and while raids continued they were scattershot and did little to dampen the growing national consensus that marijuana's medical use was incontrovertible. By the time Barak Obama assumed the presidency in 2008 there were at least eight states with medical marijuana laws on the books. Business was thriving and the focus was shifting squarely to the medical cannabis user—the patient.

Product development—which initially seemed to follow the course charted by recreational users—shifted to the patient's perspective. The first signs were in the realm of "hardware" as bongs were replaced by vaporizers—often elaborate machines that provided therapeutic dosing without the harsh, and potentially dangerous, elements of smoke inhalation.

Others reached into the past and began to re-create the tinctures and salves of old. Early 20th Century formularies were scoured for tincture "recipes" but these modern elixirs were far more sophisticated than their ancestors because modern cannabis chemists possessed the equipment to prepare carefully measured doses with specific THC and other cannabinoid content. This

proved a boon for patients who could more carefully titrate their medical intake of cannabis and, for the most part, avoid the psychoactive effects that had made the plant so notorious.

Edibles also evolved with dozens of companies creating cookies, brownies, candies and beverages, all with carefully measured dosing of cannabinoids. These products were useful for patients who needed long-term dosing of cannabis but consuming cannabis was still a tricky process. Cannabis remains an erratic substance when consumed. Individual levels of absorption can vary from day-to-day making a consistent dosing routine almost impossible. Edible cannabis products confounded the problem with packaging that was often too similar to its non-cannabis counter-parts leading to complaints that children could confuse Dad's cannabis medicine with desirable snacks.

American adults also have problems with limiting their consumption of anything that looks like a snack and parsing a cannabis-laced brownie into 4-6 dosing nibbles proved problematic for many. For those with medical needs, this form of packaging has numerous problems and states with medical cannabis laws are clamping down on edibles.

Entrepreneurs also invented some wholly new methods of cannabis administration. Chief among these is the transdermal patch. Similar to the well-known nicotine patch, cannabis transdermal patches are applied to the skin and provide a dose-related means of long-term administration that is tailor-made for many cannabis patients. Technology allows for these patches to be infused with specific cannabinoids—THC (Sativa and Indica), CBD, CBC, THCA—which allows for careful titration and maximum efficacy.

Still another innovative therapeutic innovation is a "cannabis bath salts" mixture that can be highly effective for individuals with psoriasis and other skin conditions that can be effectively treated with cannabis.

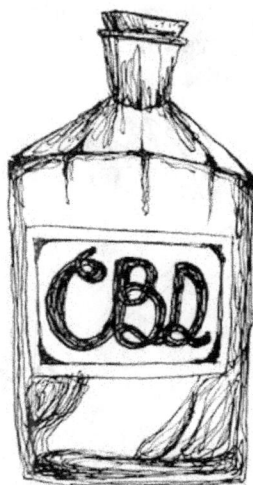

PROFESSOR DAVID PENNINGTON OF AUSTRALIA PUT IT WELL,

Cannabis can never be a pharmaceutical agent in the usual sense for medical prescription, as it contains a variety of components of variable potency and actions, depending on its origin, preparation and route of administration. Consequently, cannabis has variable effects in individuals. It will not be possible to determine universally safe dosage of cannabis for individuals based on a clinical trial.

With this mode of thinking it might be easier for the patient when he or she confronts the modern cannabis dispensary with its rows of cannabis varieties and products. Health food and supplemental stores are much the same with dizzying varieties of Omega-3 pills, oils and powder. Some may work, others may not. As the consumer we need to find the right type of cannabis to supplement our body. It won't be as easy as "take-one-pill-twice-a-day." It requires some motivation and thought from the patient and/or caregiver. It may be a new experience and it may take a while before you find "your dose."

There is a saying, "Everything old is new again." Cannabis has a long and distinguished history that for reasons of racism and economic gain was trampled on and nearly relegated to the trash bin. That dark period of our American history seems to be moving into the past and cannabis is "new again." How lucky we are to have this venerable plant back in our armamentarium of healthful, therapeutic substances. ✹

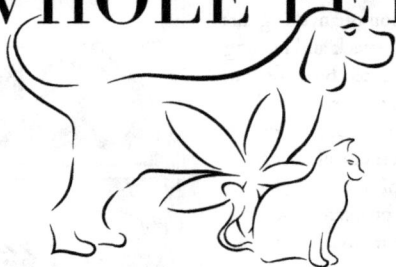

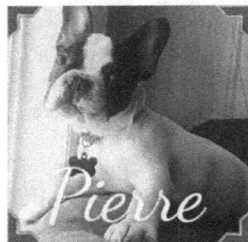

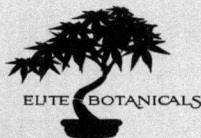

NOTES: _____

Updates for Issue #1

Graham Sorkin was Communications Director for Mary's Medicinals, 2014-2016.

Dr. Noel Palmer was Chief Scientist for Mary's Medicinals, 2014-2017.

Mary's Pets is now Mary's Whole Pet. Visit them at www.maryswholepet.com.

NOTES: _____

Mary's

CANNABIS PRIMER

issue #2

CANNABIS & CANCER

Cannabis & Cancer
Cannabis Use for Pediatric Cancers
Bobby & His Kids: Portrait of an Activist
Jonah's Story
The Bud Tender is NOT a Doctor
Industry Collaboration Helps to Educate and Empower
Patients
Interested in Exploring Cannabinoid Therapy
What is Cannabis Oil?
Legally Available Cannabis-Like Medicines
Cannabis Man

EDITOR'S NOTE

Welcome to Issue #2 of Mary's Cannabis Primer. In this issue we are focused on cannabis and cancer, in particular a broad look at the use of cannabis in treatment of pediatric cancer.

From its earliest days the medical cannabis issue has been driven by the plant's usefulness in treating the side-effects of cancer chemotherapy including emesis (nausea and vomiting) and pain. More recently there have been reports of the plant's ability to destroy cancer cells. In short, the use of cannabis in the treatment of cancer and its side-effects is at the vanguard of medical cannabis reform and will likely remain so.

Few people are aware that one patient in particular, young Danny Grinspoon, helped set the course of one of the movement's top reformers. Danny's father, Dr. Lester Grinspoon, is professor emeritus at Harvard University and author of multiple books on cannabis including the seminal, *Marihuana Reconsidered*, first released in 1971. Danny was undergoing chemotherapy in the early-1970s for acute lymphocytic leukemia (ALL), a blood cancer that often strikes children under the age of 15. Danny was diagnosed at the age of ten and grinding his way through what would be unsuccessful chemotherapy treatments when he and his mother heard rumors that other young cancer patients were using marijuana to stop the debilitating nausea and vomiting caused by Danny's chemotherapy. They were able to "score" some marijuana and it was useful to Danny but he lost his fight in 1973.

In 1978 it was a young cancer patient, Lynn Pierson, who lobbied single-handedly to pass the nation's first medical cannabis law in New Mexico. Lynn's powerful story of using marijuana to combat the nausea and vomiting associated with his chemotherapy resonated with the citizens of New Mexico and eventually the entire country. Other cancer patients in 33 states followed Pierson's lead and gave compelling testimony that led to passage of legislation recognizing the medical utility of cannabis and establishing a program of state-wide research for cancer and glaucoma patients. Few of those programs ever got started and the federal government released synthetic delta-9 THC, Marinol, to appease cancer patients and doctors. But Marinol, for most patients, is not as effective as the whole plant and today most cancer patients continue to use cannabis, normally with the complete knowledge and approval of their oncologist.

Today the focus is more on the ability of cannabinoids to destroy cancer cells. There is definite promise in the area, as Justin Kander's article (page 6) in this issue highlights. But we are a long way from being able to competently or confidently say that cannabis kills cancer. So what is a cancer patient to think or do? Dr. Grinspoon, a cancer victim himself, offers the best advice in an interview with Anthony Wile from 2014 at *The Daily Bell* (www.thedailybell.com):

> I'm afraid that people hear the statement "marijuana cures cancer" and some people are so afraid of cancer and having it treated properly by a well-qualified oncologist that they'll go right to the cannabis and say, "I'm going to treat it myself with cannabis." That's very troublesome because some of those people might have been saved or their lives prolonged if they had actually gone and gotten the best that modern Western medicine has to offer. Allopathic medicine has a long ways to go with cancer but at least some can be cured and in some, life can be prolonged quite well. I'm afraid when people think ... "Yes, marijuana cures cancer." My view is, use cannabis when you're getting the cancer treatments but [at the] first, as soon as it's diagnosed, start the treatment which medical science says is the best treatment for that but take marijuana right along. It will go much easier for you."

This question--whether cannabis should be used as an adjunct or single medication-- is obviously of vital importance to anyone using cannabis medically but perhaps even more so to the cancer patient and his or her family. In the article "Cannabis Use for Pediatric Cancers" by Dr. Bonni Goldstein (page 9) you will read first-hand accounts of both approaches. Patrick Allen (page 14) offers the perspective of a parent faced with these difficult questions and "Bobby's Kids" tells the story of one man who put his freedom on the line to help pediatric cancer patients obtain cannabis oil that would most definitely improve the quality of their life and might very well save it. Lastly, Graham Sorkin offers the perspective of a cannabis manufacturer as to where and how patients should get medical information about cannabis.

Alice O'Leary-Randall
Executive Editor - Mary's Cannabis Primer
alice@marysmedicinals.com

CANNABIS & CANCER

By Justin Kander

The use of cannabis to treat the symptoms of cancer and side-effects of chemotherapy are well known. The analgesic, neuroprotective, and stress-relieving properties of cannabis makes it the perfect tool for improving quality of life for cancer patients. Robust scientific evidence has completely confirmed the utility of cannabis for these purposes.

A 2013 trial examined 43 patients with cancer-related pain unresponsive to opiates who used a cannabis extract spray *(http://1.usa.gov/1NAMRti)*. The extract contained equal quantities of THC and CBD. On average, there were improvements in the overall level of pain severity as well as a reduction in "worst pain" levels. Insomnia and fatigue levels were also reduced, indicating better quality of life. Importantly, there was no loss of efficacy with long-term use. A double-blind, placebo-controlled trial conducted in 2014 indicated that the same THC:CBD spray helped reduce chemotherapy-induced neuropathic pain in some patients *(http://1.usa.gov/1TmPKuI)*.

A synthetic form of THC known as nabilone is approved by the FDA for treatment of chemotherapy-induced nausea and vomiting. A review study of the research found it was effective for these purposes as well as managing neuropathic pain *(http://1.usa.gov/1OCeZHm)*.

It has become apparent that whole-plant cannabis formulations are more effective than isolated, synthetic cannabinoids like nabilone. Dr. Raphael Mechoulam, who discovered THC in 1964, has posited the concept of an "entourage effect" – all the hundreds of cannabinoids and terpenes in the cannabis plant work together to provide more powerful benefits than any single compound alone *(http://cnn.it/1U2fbEh)*. Patients report better relief and less adverse side effects when using whole-plant cannabis than isolated THC *(http://bit.ly/1Xn2jv2)*. THC by itself possesses strong psychoactive properties that can cause dysphoria and other adverse effects. However, when used in lower doses with other cannabinoids like CBD, the negative effects are tempered while the positive effects are enhanced. Non-THC cannabinoids along with other therapeutic components of cannabis provide the best experiences for patients.

The most exciting aspect of using cannabis for cancer is its potential to directly kill cancer cells and inhibit growth. Since 1975, dozens of studies have been published illuminating the mechanisms by which cannabis fights cancer. The first showed how THC could slow the growth of a specific type of lung cancer *(http://1.usa.gov/1OQbMcT)*.

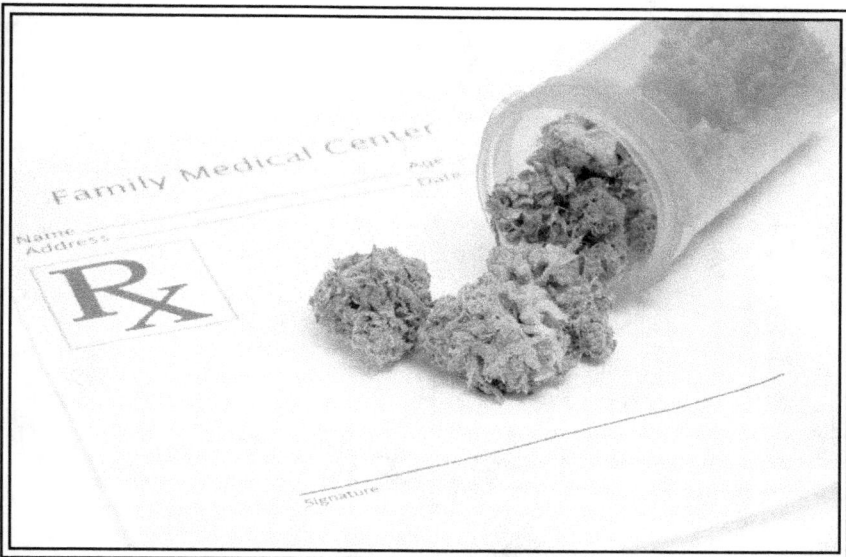

Over time, four distinct anticancer mechanisms of cannabinoids were clearly illuminated by the research. Most powerfully, they cause apoptosis, or programmed cell death, in cancer cells by activating cannabinoid receptors like CB1 and CB2 on the surface of the cells. Cannabinoids also activate other types of receptors besides the classical CB1 and CB2 receptors in order to induce apoptosis, which helps contribute to their effectiveness even in tumors expressing low levels of cannabinoid receptors. Such non-cannabinoid receptors include TRPV1 and PPAR-gamma. Cannabinoids can stop the spread, or metastasis, of cancer through several methods. For example, CBD downregulates a gene called Id-1 that is involved in promoting the metastasis of cancer. It is often cancer metastasis that makes the disease so deadly, so being able to inhibit this process is a critical attribute of any anticancer therapy.

The other major attribute of cancer is rapid, uncontrolled proliferation. All the major cannabinoids, including THC, CBD, CBN, CBC, and CBG, stop the proliferation of cancer cells. They primarily block the progression of the mitotic cell cycle, which prevents the cells from synthesizing new DNA and reproducing.

For solid tumors to grow, they require their own blood supply. They achieve this by manufacturing blood vessels, a process known as angiogenesis, to supply themselves with oxygen and nutrients. Without these dedicated blood vessels, most tumors can only grow so large. Both THC and CBD can interfere with the angiogenesis process, thus limiting the growth potential of tumors.

to receive orphan drug designation for their product than full-fledged FDA approval, there still needs to be legitimate supporting evidence. Therefore, the fact that the FDA granted CBD orphan drug status for treating glioma is a testament to the cannabinoid's very real potential for killing cancer in humans. 🍃

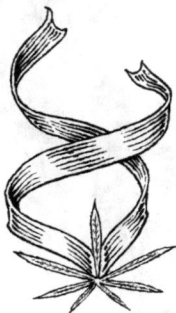

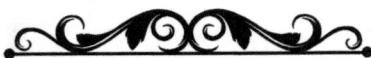

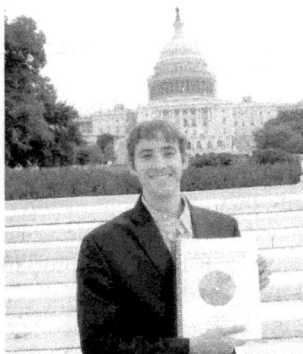

THC, CBD, and other cannabinoids have been shown in scientific studies to induce apoptosis or impair proliferation, metastasis, or angiogenesis in brain, breast, colon, liver, lung, pancreatic, prostate, and skin cancer cells, as well as leukemia, lymphoma, and other rare forms of cancer like cholangiocarcinoma and rhabdomyosarcoma. Furthermore, our own self-made endocannabinoids like anandamide kill or inhibit cancer cells through similar mechanisms as plant-based cannabinoids, such as by activating cannabinoid receptors. This phenomenon makes it far more likely the anticancer effects of THC and CBD would work in humans.

These anticancer properties are being taken very seriously by the government. A page on the National Cancer Institute's website details the antitumor properties of cannabinoids *(http://1. usa.gov/22hwq86)*. More importantly, a synthetic form of CBD is actually designated as an orphan drug by the FDA for the direct treatment of glioma brain tumors in humans *(http:// on.mktw.net/22hwB3l)*. Orphan drugs are compounds intended to treat diseases affecting 200,000 people or less, and while it is easier for a company

Justin Kander

Justin Kander has been an activist for the use of cannabis extract medicine since 2008. He has written several books on cannabis medicine including *The Comprehensive Report on the Cannabis Extract Movement, Enhancing Your Endocannabinoid System,* and *Cannabis for the Treatment of Cancer.* Kander has presented at medical cannabis conferences in Australia, Costa Rica, and The United States. He now works as the Research and Development Coordinator for Aunt Zelda's, where he writes educational material and helps produce cannabis extracts for seriously ill patients in the state of California.

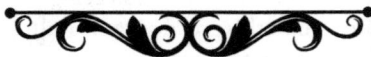

CANNABIS USE FOR PEDIATRIC CANCERS

By Bonni S. Goldstein MD

There is a tremendous amount of interest in the use of cannabis to treat cancer. Over the past two decades, hundreds of studies have investigated the antitumor properties of cannabinoids with promising results. Unfortunately we are lacking critical human research that answers the questions of which specific cancers respond to cannabis, which cannabinoids to use, what dose to use and what duration of treatment is needed to achieve survivorship.

As a pediatrician who also specializes in medical cannabis treatment, I am often asked to see children who are suffering with advanced cancers. Parents seek cannabis medicine to help their children with relief of symptoms from the adverse side effects of chemotherapy and radiation. In some cases, having been told the cancer treatment is not working, parents are desperate to find a cure. I teach parents what we know and what we don't know about cannabis use in cancer patients and in children, knowing that they must have the data to make an informed decision. Cannabinoids have been shown in animal studies to inhibit tumor growth, cause cancer cells to commit suicide, inhibit metastasis and inhibit angiogenesis (growth of new blood vessels).[1] There is only one study in humans that used THC in nine patients with unresponsive glioblastoma multiforme.[2] Human trials are prohibited in the U.S. due to the Schedule I designation of cannabis. Multiple animal studies tell us that cannabinoids have anti-proliferative effects in various tumor cell lines including breast, prostate, skin, neural, bone, and thyroid. Lymphoma and leukemia cells have also responded to cannabinoids in the lab. Additionally cannabinoids have also been shown to enhance effects of certain chemotherapeutic agents.[3,4,5] This growing evidence has triggered the use of cannabis to treat cancer in states with medical cannabis laws.

Although most reports of cancer "cures" are anecdotal, a case report from Canada of a 14-year-old girl with an extremely aggressive form of leukemia successfully documented a dose response to cannabis oil. Chemotherapy, radiation and bone marrow transplant were unsuccessful and physicians determined there was no further treatment available. The patient's parents began treating her with untested concentrated cannabis oil. The patient started treatment with a blast cell count (leukemia cells) of 194,000 (there should be none). By Day 5 of the oil, her blast cell count grew to a dangerously high 374,000, however with continued administration of the oil, by Day 15 her blast cell count was down to 61,000.

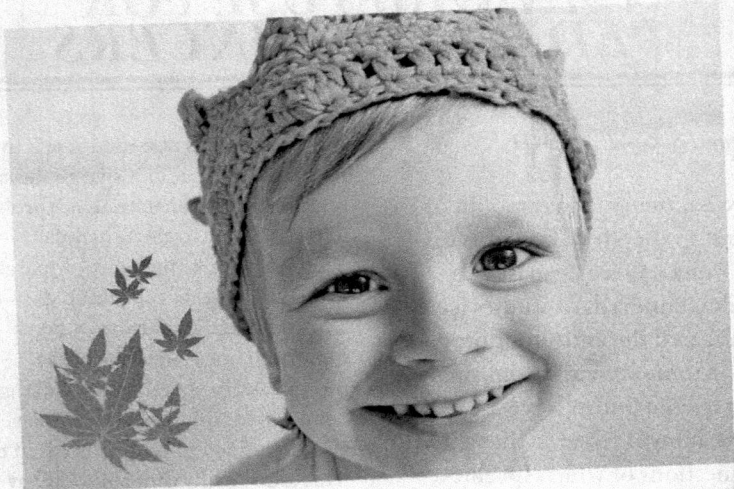

Additionally the patient required less painkillers and had increased alertness. The lowest blast cell count noted was 300 on Day 39. Ultimately the child succumbed to a bowel perforation that resulted from her severely debilitated health after 34 months of chemotherapy and radiation. During oil treatment, it was learned that blast cells increased if the oil was not taken three times/day or if a new batch was started, suggesting that longer dosing intervals and lower potency oil were less effective. This patient was not on other treatment while using cannabis and the blast cell count responded to adjustments in dosing frequency and dose potency.[6]

I am currently taking care of a teenager who was diagnosed two years ago with osteosarcoma with lung metastasis. She has been treated quite aggressively with chemotherapy and multiple surgeries.

When her parents brought her to see me, she had lost a large amount of weight, was in terrible pain and was on palliative chemotherapy of gemcitabine. The oncologist reported to me that there was no further treatment available. The patient was started on a regimen of high dose THC and CBD oil sublingually, starting low doses and ultimately increasing to 1000 mg cannabinoids/day divided in three doses with a 1:1 CBD:THC ratio with instructions to continue chemo. She immediately gained weight and stopped using opiates for pain. After three months of cannabis treatment, repeat bone and PET scans revealed no evidence of disease. The patient continued on cannabis treatment but due to development of anxiety, the CBD:THC ratio was adjusted to 3:1. After another three months of oil treatment, repeat radiological evaluation revealed no evidence of disease. The patient is still on cannabis and is awaiting the next round of scans. She is back in school and living her life. What is notable in this case is that research in mice with grafted pancreatic cancer cells showed that the gemcitabine's ability to kill cancer cells was enhanced by the addition of cannabinoids.[7] I believe that the synergy between the chemo and cannabinoids is the reason why this young girl is in remission.

Cannabis treatment for children with cancer remains controversial, however in cases of treatment-resistant cancers and severe side effects from treatment, cannabis must be a readily available option, especially since it is significantly less toxic than most cancer treatments. In addition to the antitumor effects, cannabis can enhance the effects of some chemotherapy while making the adverse effects tolerable. In my experience, I have seen patient survival extended. We must be careful with claims of "cancer cure" but if cannabis can be rescheduled from Schedule I to Schedule II, researchers can finally find the desperately needed answers and save many lives. ❦

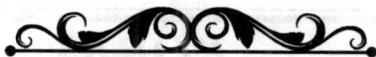

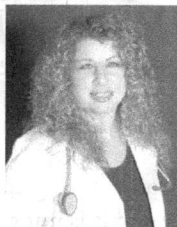

Bonni S. Goldstein MD

A native of New Jersey, Dr. Bonni Goldstein received her undergraduate education at Rutgers College and pursued her medical degree at Robert Wood Johnson Medical School at the University of Medicine and Dentistry of New Jersey. Her post-doctoral education included internship and residency at Children's Hospital Los Angeles. Dr. Goldstein also served as Chief Resident at Children's Hospital Los Angeles. She was a Clinical Instructor in Pediatrics at USC School of Medicine in Los Angeles, Emergency Transport Attending Physician at Children's Hospital Los Angeles and Emergency Medicine Attending Physician in the Pediatric Emergency Department at Los Angeles County-USC Medical Center. In 2008, Dr. Goldstein developed an interest in the science of medical cannabis after witnessing its beneficial effects in an ill friend. Since then she has been evaluating both adult and pediatric patients for use of medical cannabis.

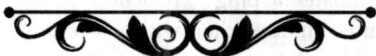

Sources:
1. **Zogopoulos, Panagiotis, et al.** "The antitumor action of cannabinoids on glioma tumorigenesis." Histology & Histopathology 30 (2015).
2. **Guzman, M., et al.** "A pilot clinical study of Δ9-tetrahydrocannabinol in patients with recurrent glioblastoma multiforme." British journal of cancer 95.2 (2006): 197-203.
3. **Miyato, Hideyo, et al.** "Pharmacological synergism between cannabinoids and paclitaxel in gastric cancer cell lines." Journal of Surgical Research 155.1 (2009): 40-47.
4. **Nabissi, Massimo, et al.** "Triggering of the TRPV2 channel by cannabidiol sensitizes glioblastoma cells to cytotoxic chemotherapeutic agents." Carcinogenesis 34.1 (2013): 48-57.
5. **Donadelli, M., et al.** "Gemcitabine/cannabinoid combination triggers autophagy in pancreatic cancer cells through a ROS-mediated mechanism." Cell death & disease 2.4 (2011): e152
6. **Singh, Yadvinder, and Chamandeep Bali.** "Cannabis extract treatment for terminal acute lymphoblastic leukemia with a Philadelphia chromosome mutation." Case reports in oncology 6.3 (2013): 585-592.)
7. **Donadelli, M., et al.** "Gemcitabine/cannabinoid combination triggers autophagy in pancreatic cancer cells through a ROS-mediated mechanism." Cell death & disease 2.4 (2011): e152.

BOBBY & HIS KIDS: PORTRAIT OF AN ACTIVIST

By Alice O'Leary-Randall

Nothing is quite as tragic as a child with cancer and it is not surprising that people are drawn to help these children. Bobby Moulton is one of those people. The soft-spoken, Indiana native loves kids and a few years back he found his calling when he learned how effective cannabis oil could be in the treatment of cancer, particularly pediatric cancer.

"I was a sick 'lil one myself," he recalls. "Ear infections, pneumonia, seizures and a bleeding ulcer that perforated when I was 13. I became involved with sick kids at birth."

Moulton decided to devote his life to helping pediatric cancer patients and estimates helping 35 patients directly and countless others with advice and guidance. In the summer of 2014, he moved to Rhode Island, a legal cannabis state, to be closer a young boy he was helping in New York. That fall, Moulton was arrested for marijuana.

His arrest was the result of a betrayal by a 20-year-old Michigander whom Moulton refers to as "the kid" and whom he agreed to help by giving the young man a new start in Rhode Island. While Moulton was away in Ohio "the kid" stole Moulton's cannabis oil and sold it to some real kids in the town of West Warwick. A 13-year-old girl became ill and police arrested "the kid" who copped a plea and turned in Moulton. The police seized 4-5 ounces of trim, 4-6 plants, 60 grams of oil, syringes and empty capsules. But what really nailed Moulton was the "still" that he used to manufacture the cannabis oil. He was charged with manufacturing with intent to sell.

"I drove back from Ohio to turn myself in thinking I would go in and out fast. I have a very good legal team, "Moulton explained. "That was not the case. They held me two weeks."

When Moulton finally was released on bail he returned to an eviction notice at his apartment and everything of any value was gone. His lawyer told him, solemnly, he was facing decades in jail. Rhode Island is one of 23 states that recognizes the medical utility of cannabis. The law was passed in 2005 and allows possession of 2.5 usable ounces and up to 12 plants for patients. Moulton hoped to become a registered caregiver in the state which would have allowed up to 5 ounces and 24 plants but he had not yet fulfilled the residency requirement for the state. Regardless, Moulton was in clear violation of the state medical cannabis regulations.

"If I have to take it for the kids," he said a few months after his arrest with a mixture of bravura and resignation, "Then, that's what I'll do."

Thankfully that will not be the case Moulton appealed to his friends and clients for help. The mothers of 25 children helped by Moulton's cannabis oil sent letters to Judge Joseph A. Montalbano, pleading with the judge to go easy on the Indiana native who took the stand on his own behalf despite some concerns that it could backfire. Afterwards Moulton's attorney, Victor Baretta, who had advised Moulton to expect a minimum sentence of five years, told his client that the testimony was, "F@!king epic!" Moulton's modest reply to such praise was, "It's not hard to be convincing when you're telling the truth." The judge seemed moved by his testimony, stating, with a confused shake of the head, "In some way you seem to feel this is honorable."

Well, yes, Bobby Moulton does... and so do lots of other people. When asked what his plans are now, Bobby replied, "Keep on keeping on. The kids still need me." 🌿

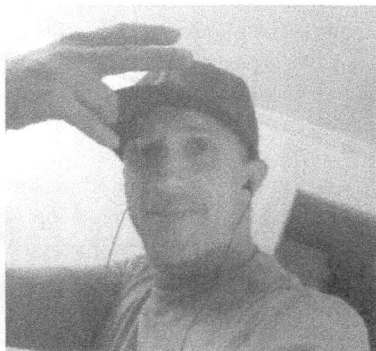

WHAT ARE THE DIFFERENCES BETWEEN CANCERS IN ADULTS AND CHILDREN?

The types of cancers that develop in children are often different from the types that develop in adults. Childhood cancers are often the result of DNA changes in cells that take place very early in life, sometimes even before birth. Unlike many cancers in adults, childhood cancers are not strongly linked to lifestyle or environmental risk factors.

There are exceptions, but childhood cancers tend to respond better to treatments such as chemotherapy. Children's bodies also tend to tolerate chemotherapy better than adults' bodies do. But cancer treatments such as chemotherapy and radiation therapy can have some long-term side effects, so children who survive their cancer need careful attention for the rest of their lives.

Courtesy of the American Cancer Society web page:
http://www.cancer.org/cancer/neuroblastoma/detailedguide/neuroblastoma-differences-children-adults

JONAH'S STORY

By Patrick Allen

It was mid November 2012, just under two months after we moved our family from Colorado to New England, and we were scheduled for a routine scan at Boston Children's Hospital for our 2 year-old son Jonah because he has hydrocephalus (an abnormal accumulation of fluids in the brain). This was our chance to meet Jonah's new Neurosurgeon and let the doc get a baseline scan of Jonah's brain. This was also our first trip to Boston since moving and we were really excited to get to the big city.

During the scan a growth was noticed and soon we were sitting in an old New England office building connected to the hospital. The doc delivered the news, "Were you guys aware of the growth on Jonah's brain." My wife and I couldn't believe our ears. "What do you mean? What kind of growth? Is it cancer?" A million questions went through our heads. The doc told us that the tumor was most likely a glioma and could be low grade. Still, low grade, high grade, didn't matter. Tumors can grow fast or slow unexpectedly at any time. And this one was inoperable: directly on the thalamus. Over the next few weeks we met with the Oncology department and while Boston Children's has a tremendous team we still had very few answers. After discussing

the circumstances and Jonah's past, it was decided to watch the tumor for 3 months before taking next steps---biopsy, chemo and then radiation. All are super dangerous and all take a massive toll on the body.

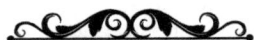

> *I found government documentation showing the U.S. government held a patent for cannabis oil as a cure for cancer*

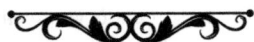

In the meantime, I could not help but look into every possible solution for my son's recovery and health. As I was doing this research, my brother (who, by the way, spent years in my youth convincing me to quit smoking pot, which I finally did) brought up something super interesting. He asked if I knew anything about cannabis oil. He said he read an article about a dad in Montana who gave his son cannabis oil and saw amazing results. I found the article and was extremely moved. I spent the following days/weeks doing nothing but praying, research, and talking to people to get their wisdom. I created a second Facebook page to connect with people using cannabis oil so I wouldn't have the judgment of my current "friends"

on Facebook. I found so many families using the oil and having great success. And I found government documentation showing the U.S. government held a patent for cannabis oil as a cure for cancer--more specifically, brain tumors/gliomas. I was beside myself. How could I take my son from the very best pediatric oncology center in the world and use cannabis oil? Besides, it wasn't accessible in New England at a level that we needed if we wanted to try it.

I contacted The Realm of Caring back in Colorado. I reached out to them and they offered a ton of wisdom, guidance and assured a good, reliable, clean source of oil. The thought of moving back to Colorado was daunting and scary to say the least. Would my job let me come back? Where would we live? What would the docs at Boston Children's think?

How everything fell together was a God thing. I don't know how else to put it. Boston Children's Hospital advised watching it for 3 months. My job was more than willing to let me come back to Colorado. I called some friends from high school who own The Green Solution, a dispensary in Colorado, and they were excited to start a fundraiser for Jonah. The Realm of Caring had everything in place for us the get access to cannabis oil in Colorado. And we somehow found a rental home that was perfect for us. In fact, I was driving our moving truck back west and was 15 min away from meeting up with my wife at her aunt and uncle's where we were going to stay until we could get a place when the landlord called and said "I had over 30 applicants and yours was the best, you

can move in tomorrow." This happened to be Christmas Eve.

We were able to start Jonah's oil by early January and the follow up scan in early March already showed the tumor had shrunk. Jonah has been on cannabis oil for almost two years now and every scan shows the tumor smaller and less alive looking.

Moving across country and not having accessibility made things extremely difficult. Even today, we cannot go on an out-of-state vacation and still give Jonah the oil he needs. But at the end of the day, we are just so thankful that we have access where we are and for all of the people and organizations that have made it possible! 🌿

WHAT ARE THE MOST COMMON TYPES OF CHILDHOOD CANCERS?

The types of cancers that occur most often in children are different from those seen in adults. The most common cancers of children are:

- **Leukemia** (a cancer of the blood)
- **Brain and other central nervous system tumors**
- **Neuroblastoma** (a cancer of immature nerve cells, particularly in an embryo and fetus)
- **Wilms tumor** (a type of kidney cancer in children)
- **Lymphoma** (including both Hodgkin and non-Hodgkin. A cancer of the lymph glands.)
- **Rhabdomyosarcoma** (a cancer of the cells that normally develop into skeletal muscles)
- **Retinoblastoma** (a cancer of the eye)
- **Bone cancer** (including osteosarcoma and Ewing sarcoma)

Other types of cancers are rare in children, but they do happen sometimes. In very rare cases, children may even develop cancers that are much more common in adults.

THE BUD TENDER IS _NOT_ A DOCTOR

By Graham Sorkin

There are wonderful stories about patients with a multitude of different disorders whose lives have been transformed by the use of medical cannabis. But for a cannabis naïve or newly diagnosed patient the pressing question is – _"Where do I start?"_

One of the biggest challenges in medical cannabis today is the lack of reliable information about how to actually use it. Normally a patient will ask their doctor or nurse about treatment options but with cannabis it is often a friend, hip grandchild or a friendly bud tender.

As an infused product manufacturer, I am frequently put in the position of being asked for medical advice. Putting aside the fact that it would be unethical for me to provide such advice, I'm concerned that these patients are coming to me instead of their doctors or care specialists. I'm not a doctor. I cannot and should not dispense medical advice.

I can tell you all about how products are made, how cannabinoids in our products interact with the body's endocannabinoid system, and how we ensure the quality of products we offer—but I am certainly not the right person to tell you how to treat dystonia, cancer, arthritis or any number of other ailments.

People are often willing to take huge risks by changing their medical-care regimens without proper supervision, especially patients facing a life-threatening disease. The friendly bud tender who offers promising anecdotal advice--"You don't need chemo, just load up on CBD. It worked for this guy I know."—may think the information is helpful but they do not have sufficient expertise to make such a claim.

If that patient's health takes a turn for the worse and their family blames the bud tender for suggesting alternative treatment, it will spell trouble for not just that individual or dispensary but for our industry as a whole.

> "It's still unconventional and doesn't fit neatly into the 'take-one-pill-twice-a-day' model to which Westerners are accustomed."

No medicine works for everyone. Despite some exciting research in the past decade we understand a lot less about how cannabis works than many other modern medicines. It's still unconventional and doesn't fit neatly into the "take-one-pill-twice-a-day" model to which Westerners are accustomed. That's why it is more difficult to prescribe than most other treatments.

As a community, our task is to ensure that patients understand the vast potential of cannabis medicine, and just as importantly, understand that they need to have a clear, honest conversation with qualified medical providers about if and how they will use it. With a small but growing body of knowledge, grass-roots nonprofit groups such as Realm of Caring have taken it upon themselves to start Institutional Review Board (IRB)-approved observational-research studies that gather information and enable patients to actively contribute data about their experiences to help others more effectively use cannabis medicine.

But we need more options for medical providers to learn about the rapidly advancing field of cannabinoid medicine and more professionals that are informed about cannabis to share their knowledge. Similarly, dispensary owners and employees owe it to their customers to become educated about the complex and promising world of cannabis therapeutics. We applaud groups such as the American Cannabis Nurses Association and Patients Out of Time that host ongoing educational events for medical professionals and reformers. Now let's ensure that all of our care providers know about these groups and take advantage of the resources they provide. We know there are small communities of doctors, nurses and care providers that understand how to safely use these treatments. The next step is helping them create larger networks to share their findings and research to benefit all of us.

Anyone who has spent any time talking with people in the cannabis industry knows that cannabinoid therapy has incredible potential for healing. Everyone involved is enthusiastically trying to get these treatments into the hands of anyone who could benefit. However, we can't let excitement and compassion overwhelm common sense or we risk the validity and longevity of the movement. ❧

INDUSTRY COLLABORATION HELPS TO EDUCATE AND EMPOWER PATIENTS INTERESTED IN EXPLORING CANNABINOID THERAPY

Mary's Medicinals & Nutritionals Teams with Realm of Caring to provide Support Services and Resources for Those Using Cannabinoid Products

Mary's Medicinals recently announced that it has teamed with Realm of Caring to fund research, education and patient empowerment efforts both locally in Colorado and nationwide. As part of the partnership, Realm of Caring's extensive client support resources are now available to all Mary's Medicinals and Mary's Nutritionals customers.

The Realm of Caring is a 501(c)(3) non-profit organization that provides a better quality of life for those affected by disorders and diseases, including but not limited to, Cancer, MS, HIV/AIDS, Epilepsy and Parkinson's through the use of cannabinoid products. Each client's progress is monitored through an Institutional Review Board (IRB) approved observational research study. Through these studies, the Realm of Caring is able to educate the general public as to the benefits and effects of cannabinoid supplements.

"We're continuing to see the potential of the cannabis plant to change people's lives," said Nicole Smith, founder & CEO of Mary's Medicinals, Mary's Nutritionals and Mary's Pets. "The challenge today is the limited availability of reliable research, information, and support. Realm of Caring is leading the charge to educate patients and their families.

We're honored to be involved in their mission and excited to help make these critical resources available to more patients."

The Realm of Caring Foundation was established in 2012 by The Stanley Brothers, Heather Jackson, and Paige Figi — following the first two success stories of their children using Charlotte's Web™.

"For some, cannabinoid products may offer their only chance for relief," said Heather Jackson, Executive Director, Realm of Caring. "Through ongoing research projects, RoC is becoming an educational resource for consumers, physicians, scientists, governments and the media. We're excited to team with Mary's to support families and medical professionals worldwide." 🌿

CONTACT REALM OF CARING:

719-347-5400
theroc.us

WHAT IS CANNABIS OIL?

We asked Mary's Medicinals chief scientist, Dr. Noel Palmer, just what is Cannabis Oil?

Cannabis 'oils' or 'concentrates' are produced by collecting cannabinoids from the surface of the plant either by physical or chemical means. These cannabinoids (e.g. THC, CBD, etc) are found in the trichomes—the hairy protrusions which are present on the surface of the plant's leaves. Modern photography has revealed the beauty of these integral cannabis components and these can be viewed online by simply searching for "cannabis trichome images." Physical methods to collect these cannabinoids (for example, scraping the leaves) will produce what's commonly referred to as 'hash' and/or 'kief'. This method is effective but, obviously has some drawbacks. For example, simply scraping the leaves will also collect residual plant matter which lowers the total potency.

Chemical methods used to collect cannabinoids might include: alcohols (e.g. ethanol), hydrocarbons (e.g. butane) or supercritical CO_2. Common names for chemically derived concentrates might include "shatter" or "wax." The concentration of cannabinoids on dry plant material can range from 1-25% of the total mass. The concentration of cannabinoids in 'concentrates' or 'oils' can average from 40% to greater than 80% depending on the methods used. Production methods can also effect the final potency of the preparation.

Producing concentrates or oils using appropriate methods and solvents is critical --- otherwise dangerous contaminants can be introduced to the final product. Store bought chemicals (e.g. from a hardware store) have been shown to be unacceptably purified to produce medicinal quality cannabis concentrates and oils.

∾ MARINOL ∽

The granddaddy of legal cannabis medicines, also called dronabinol, Marinol is synthetic delta-9 THC. The drug was originally developed by the U.S. government for use in animal experiments. It was never intended for therapeutic use but became legally available in the 1980s when the federal government released Marinol, calling it "the pot pill," in order to deflect the momentum of the growing medical marijuana movement. It is used primarily for nausea and vomiting or for appetite stimulation.

∾ CESAMET ∽

Otherwise known as nabilone. Cesamet has an interesting history in the medical cannabis battle. Developed in the 1970s by Eli Lilly, the drug was once fast-tracked by the FDA in hopes it could be

released and stifle the growing clamor for legal, medical marijuana. But in the late 1970s, long-term studies of the drug had disastrous results when beagle dogs began to spasm and then die. Eli Lilly was forced back to the drawing board and the U.S. federal government was forced to release Marinol. Today Cesamet (approved in the U.S. in 1985) is available in several countries and is used as an anti-nausea drug and also as an adjunct treatment for neuropathic pain.

∾ SATIVEX ∽

Actually derived from the cannabis plant, Sativex is manufactured by G.W. Pharmaceuticals in the United Kingdom. It is also known as nabiximols. The drug is delivered via an inhaler, which makes it fast acting. It was primarily developed for multiple sclerosis patients to combat the spasms, neuropathic pain and overactive bladder associated with that disease. It is also being investigated as a treatment for pain related to cancer. Sativex is not yet available in the U.S. but is available in 28 countries worldwide.

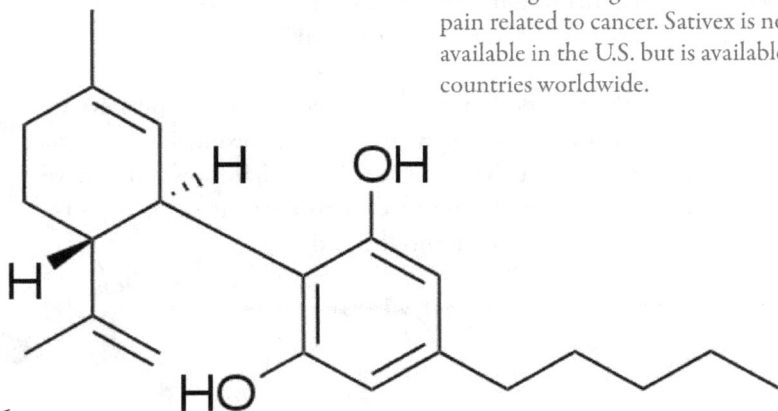

Updates for Issue #2

Graham Sorkin was Communications Director for Mary's Medicinals, 2014-2016.

Dr. Noel Palmer was Chief Scientist for Mary's Medicinals, 2014-2017.

Bobby Moulton continues working with "his kids" and lives in Indiana.

Jonah Allen is, according to his parents, "doing great! Our little boy is doing so well and he's not so little anymore. He's growing strong and playing hard. His little sister Iris is his best friend and he loves playing tag, hide and go seek and trying to run as fast as he can. While he still suffers from a gait in his walk he's giving it all he has. We have since had 2 scans for Jonah and we are seeing no changes from the last scan. What is left, does not look like much and may be only be scar tissue. For this past couple of years Jonah has been using Haleigh's Hope and Cannatol oil in much smaller doses than we originally started with. We are really pleased with where he is today and have big hopes for his future."

CANNABIS MAN

WHOLE BODY RELIEF & PROTECTION

CBD, CBG, CBC & THC
inhibit cell growth & cancer cells

CBD, CBC, CBN & THC
reduces or eliminates pain

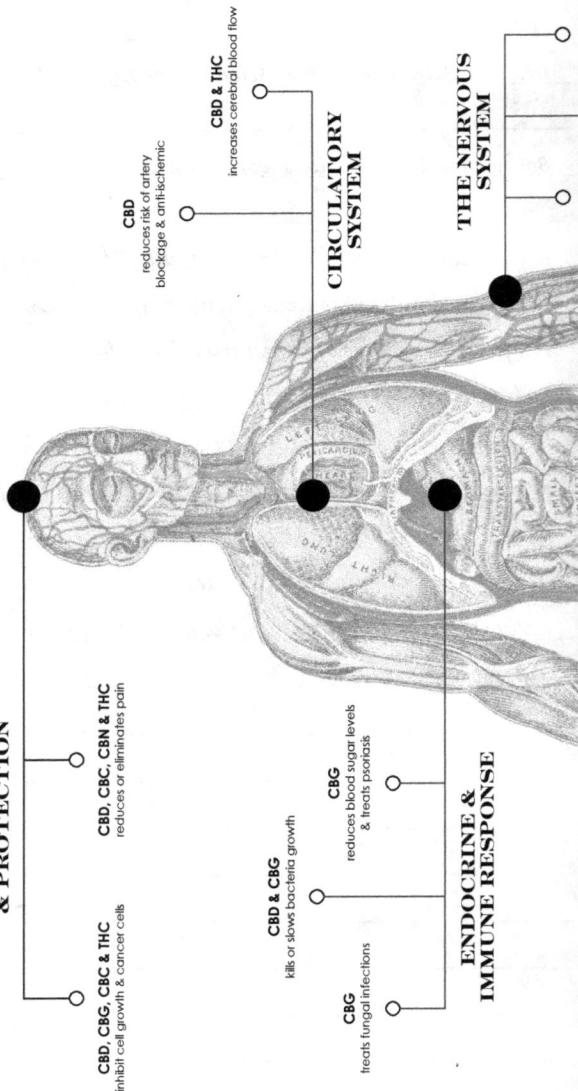

CBD & CBG
kills or slows bacteria growth

CBG
reduces blood sugar levels & treats psoriasis

CBG
treats fungal infections

ENDOCRINE & IMMUNE RESPONSE

CBD
reduces risk of artery blockage & anti-ischemic

CBD & THC
increases cerebral blood flow

CIRCULATORY SYSTEM

THE NERVOUS SYSTEM

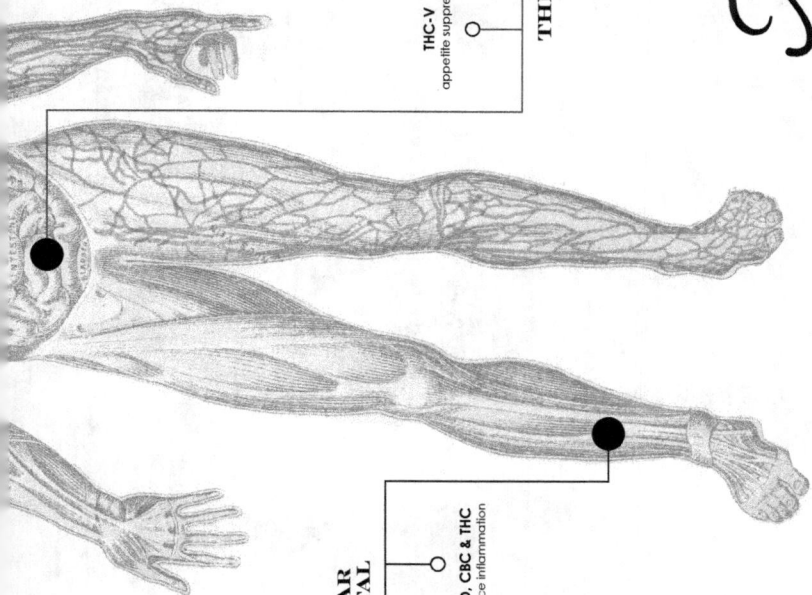

CBD
tranquilizes &
relieves anxiety

CBN
aids in sleep

CBD & THC-V
reduces seizures & convulsions

THC
appetite stimulant

CBD
reduces contractions
in the small intestines

THC-V
appetite suppressant

THE DIGESTIVE SYSTEM

MUSCULAR & SKELETAL

CBD, CBC & THC
reduce inflammation

CBD, CBN & THC
suppress muscle spasms

CBD, CBG, CBC & THC-V
promote bone health

Mary's

MEDICINALS

39

Mary's

CANNABIS PRIMER

issue #3

THE ENDOCANNABINOID SYSTEM

Chronic Pain & Medical Cannabis
The Endocannabinoid System: A Physician's Perspective
Medical Cannabis Laws Map
Here's the Thing: A Mother's Story
How to Find It: Searching for Medical Cannabis Information

EDITOR'S NOTE

An Apology to Those Who Have Been Wronged

Several decades ago, when I was a young and passionate activist just starting the fight for medical cannabis, I confess there seemed to be a lot of questionable claims made about cannabis. In 1975, my late husband, with the help of researchers at UCLA, had proven conclusively that cannabis helped his glaucoma. Reports by cancer patients that cannabis helped with the side-effects of chemotherapy were also bolstered by some research and certainly by the dramatic testimony of the patients and their families. But many other patients came forward with all kinds of ailments: multiple sclerosis, chronic pain, epilepsy, Chron's Disease, Parkinson's Disease, eczema, retinitis pigmentosa, migraines, anorexia, bipolar disorder, schizophrenia and more. How, I wondered, could cannabis help so many diverse conditions? Federal officials and physicians thought the same thing. In voices dripping with disdain and condemnation these "authorities" would declare that no drug could do everything that proponents claimed of cannabis. Intellectually it was easy to agree.

But the calls kept coming and the list of ailments helped by cannabis seemed to get longer. In the 1980s I fear that I may have been too dismissive of some patients who contacted our group, Alliance for Cannabis Therapeutics. I would listen, send information and tell many of these folks that legal access to federal supplies of cannabis via the government's Compassionate IND Program was really unlikely (it was). I would hear the disappointment in their voices and frustration that their pleas were not being heard.

In 1992, however, a discovery was made that would forever alter the medical cannabis debate. Building on the 1988 discovery of cannabinoid receptors in the human body, an Israeli research team headed by Dr. Raphael Mechoulam, put together the puzzle and announced that all mammals have an endogenous cannabinoid system (ECS). In short, our body already produces cannabinoid-like substances and has receptors for those natural cannabinoids substances as well as the phyto-cannabinoids produced in cannabis. But most remarkably it was determined that these cannabinoid-like substances assist our body with its most fundamental job—homeostasis.

Homeostasis is no small thing. It is defined as, "The tendency of the body to seek and maintain a condition of balance or equilibrium within its internal environment, even when faced with external changes." Discovery of the ECS changed our way of looking at homeostasis and has dramatically altered the research path. Today the sky seems to be the limit with respect to cannabis research and laboratories are popping with new discoveries. Their discoveries are verifying the anecdotal observations of those patients I met long ago and they are opening the door for new applications of this remarkable plant.

This issue of *Mary's Cannabis Primer* looks at the ECS and introduces our readers to this truly remarkable system that is so important to our physiological well-being. Dr. Dustin Sulak, one of the nation's pre-eminent cannabis practitioners, has provided us with an excellent article about the ECS and helps provide perspective on this important topic (page 11). Another feature article concerns cannabis and the treatment of chronic pain (page 6). Our regular features of Cannabis Man (page 24) and Selection Guide (page 8) offer readers an easy and concise summary of which cannabinoids are most helpful for which disease categories. In the article "How to Find It?", the *Primer* provides hints on how to use the internet to find additional information on the ECS, your specific disease and the use of cannabis to treat it (page 21). *The Primer* concludes with its regular first-hand account of medical cannabis use. "Here's The Thing" is written by Heather Jackson, CEO of the Realm of Caring Foundation (page 19).

Heather's moving account of treating her son Zaki with medical cannabis may sound familiar to many of our readers. The path that brings patients to medical cannabis is remarkably consistent and yet genuinely moving in each case. Desperation grows as conventional medications fail to help. There is disbelief that something as natural as cannabis can actually help but with no other available options there is nothing to lose. Acceptance of the effectiveness of cannabis eventually occurs and the patient, with his or her caregivers, is launched on a path that they never imagined. They become a part of the growing legions that demand legal access to quality-controlled cannabis medications.

It has been my honor to help expand the understanding of cannabis' medical utility. I think back on my skepticism with some of those patients whom I talked with several decades ago and I quietly say, "I'm sorry." And then I re-commit myself to this important matter of public health. Cannabis, it seems, has always been a part of mankind's existence. It is time to remove the shackles that were placed upon it in the 20th Century and resume this remarkable co-existence, unencumbered by governmental restrictions.

Alice O'Leary-Randall
Executive Editor - Mary's Cannabis Primer
alice@marysmedicinals.com
www.aliceolearyrandall.com

CHRONIC PAIN & MEDICAL CANNABIS

By: *Alice O'Leary-Randall*
Executive Editor - Mary's Cannabis Primer

Editor's Note: This article first appeared in Cannabis Now Magazine.

In the 2014 book, *A Nation in Pain*, Judy Foreman offered a stunning picture of America's growing problem with chronic pain. Tucked quietly within that volume is Chapter 10, "Marijuana: The Weed America Loves to Hate." In it Foreman concludes: "to put it bluntly, marijuana [for pain] works. Not dazzlingly, but about as well as opioids. That is, it can reduce chronic pain by more than 30 percent. And with fewer serious side effects."

The same conclusion has been reached by many Americans. *Marijuana Business Daily* recently reported that chronic pain comprised a whopping 64.2% of patients in those medical cannabis states that track a registrant's medical condition. If you apply that percentage to the estimated 100 million adults living in chronic pain (Institute of Medicine, "Relieving Pain in America," 2011) you can quickly see that nationwide availability to medical cannabis could have a profound impact on the nation's health, improve the quality of life for millions, and, not incidentally, vastly expand the medical cannabis market.

Who Can Use and Where?

Of the 27 state laws that allow medical access to cannabis, 22 specifically mention "chronic," "intractable," or "severe" pain as a qualifying condition. An additional three— Illinois, New Hampshire, and Massachusetts—give the physician sufficient leeway to recommend cannabis for pain. In Connecticut, Florida and New Jersey a patient with chronic pain must be certified as terminally ill.

Another 17 states have the so-called CBD-only laws but, in most cases, use is restricted to pediatric epilepsy patients.

The Research

Opponents of medical cannabis are quick to single out the chronic pain patient as some kind of pariah, implying that pain is an "excuse" to abuse drugs. They will say there is no research to support the use of cannabis in pain therapy when, actually, quite the opposite is true. A Google Scholar search using the exact phrase "cannabis and pain" reveals 27 studies between 2000-2016. Another 40 studies are

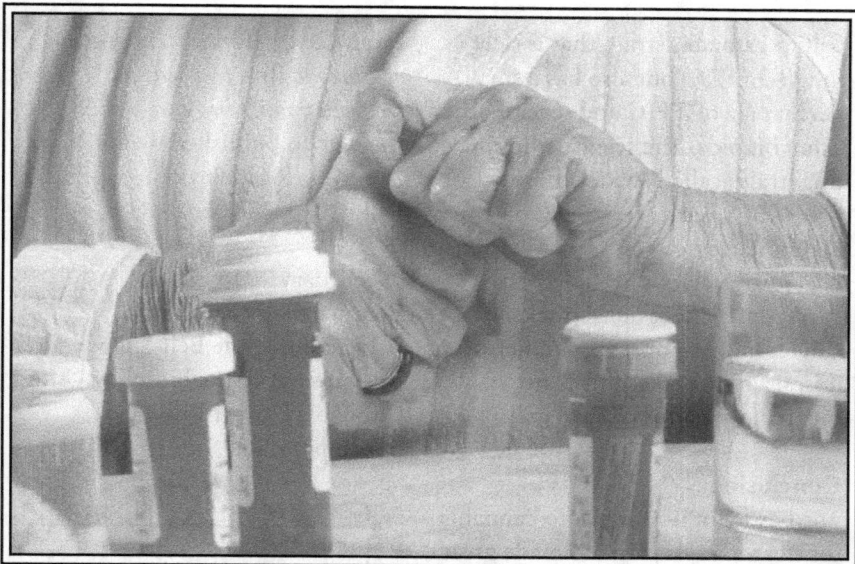

presented when the phrase is changed to "marijuana and pain."

Nearly all present a positive view of the use of cannabis in treating pain, especially neuropathic or nerve pain. A particularly thorough review prepared in 2013 for the American Academy of Pain* by Ethan Russo observes that these studies, "provide provocative direction to inform modern research on treatment of pain and other conditions, [but] it does not represent evidence ... that is commonly acceptable to governmental regulatory bodies with respect to pharmaceutical development."

And therein lies the rub. Without a pharmaceutical advocate cannabis will never win a government seal of approval for prescribed use. Current research, however, is beneficial to pharmaceutical companies seeking approval for prescribed cannabis products and it is also beneficial for the patients.

But Natural Is Better

For many the concept of cannabis parsed and packaged as a pharmaceutical product is abhorrent. They point to the well-known "entourage effect," i.e. cannabinoids work better together rather than in isolation. And their argument is backed by science. In 2015, Israeli scientists** reported findings involving synthetically produced, single molecule CBD vs. naturally occurring CBD derived from a cannabis strain that is rich in CBD (17%) but also has a small percentage of THC and several other cannabinoids. The scientists found this strain, called Avidekel, "superior over CBD for the treatment of inflammatory conditions." Synthetic CBD had a clear threshold of therapeutic effect but Avidekel has "increasing responses upon increasing doses, which makes this plant medicine ideal for clinical uses."

Conclusion

The battle for licit access to cannabis for treatment of pain has made great

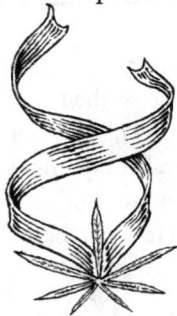

strides in the past two decades. Research supports it and common decency demands it. Judge Gustin L. Reichbach wrote in May 2012 in an op-ed piece of *The New York Times*. "When palliative care is understood as a fundamental human and medical right, marijuana for medical use should be beyond controversy." Judge Reichlich, a cancer patient, died two months later.

From *Comprehensive Treatment of Chronic Pain by Medical, Interventional, and Integrative Approaches* published by the American Academy of Pain. 2013. entitled.

** February 2015 issue of Pharmacology & Pharmacy , "Overcoming the Bell-Shaped Dose-Response of Cannabidiol by Using Cannabis Extract Enriched in Cannabidiol."

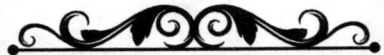

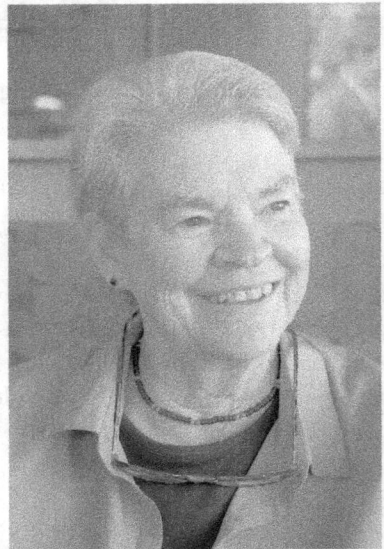

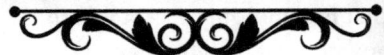

Alice O'Leary-Randall is a true medical cannabis pioneer with more than forty years in the issue. To learn more about Alice please visit: **www.aliceolearyrandall.com**

THE ENDOCANNBINOID SYSTEM: A PHYSICIAN'S PERSPECTIVE

By Dr. Dustin Sulak, D.O.
healer.com

Editor's Note: This article first appeared in the NORML publication, Emerging Clinical Applications For Cannabis & Cannabinoids, which is available online at: http://norml.org/ library/recent-research-on-medical- marijuana. Mary's Foundation thanks NORML and Dr. Sulak for giving permission to reprint.

At our integrative medical clinics in Maine and Massachusetts, my colleagues and I treat over 18,000 patients with a huge diversity of diseases and symptoms. In one day I might see cancer, Crohn's disease, epilepsy, chronic pain, multiple sclerosis, insomnia, Tourette's syndrome and eczema, just to name a few. All of these conditions have different causes, different physiologic states, and vastly different symptoms. The patients are old and young. Some are undergoing conventional therapy. Others are on a decidedly alternative path. Yet despite their differences, almost all of my patients would agree on one point: cannabis helps their condition. How is this possible?

As a physician, I am naturally wary of any medicine that purports to cure-all. Panaceas, snake-oil remedies, and expensive fads often come and go, with big claims but little scientific or clinical evidence to support their efficacy. As I explore the therapeutic potential of cannabis, however, I find no lack of evidence. In fact, I find an explosion of scientific research on the therapeutic potential of cannabis, more evidence than one can find on some of the most widely used therapies of conventional medicine.

In October 2016, a PubMed search for scientific journal articles published in the last 20 years containing the word "cannabis" revealed 10,425 results. (https:// www.ncbi.nlm.nih.gov/pubmed) Add the word "cannabinoid," and the results increase to 24,230 articles. That's an average of more than three scientific publications per day over the last 20 years! These numbers not only illustrate the present scientific interest and financial investment in understanding more about cannabis and its components, but they also emphasize the need for high quality reviews and summaries such as the document you are about to read. (Note: an excellent source for this type of information is Dr. Roger Pertwee's *Handbook of Cannabis*.)

How can one herb help so many different conditions? How can it provide both palliative and curative actions? How can it be so safe while offering such powerful effects? The search to answer these questions has led scientists to the discovery of a previously unknown physiologic system, a central component of the health and healing of every human and almost every animal: the endocannabinoid system.

What Is The Endocannabinoid System?

The endogenous cannabinoid system (ECS), named after the plant that led to its discovery, is perhaps the most important physiologic system involved in establishing and maintaining human health. Endocannabinoids and their receptors are found throughout the body: in the brain, organs, connective tissues, glands, and immune cells. In each tissue, the endocannabinoid system performs different tasks, but the goal is always the same: homeostasis— the maintenance of a stable internal physiologic environment despite fluctuations in the external environment.

Cannabinoids promote homeostasis at every level of biological life, from the sub-cellular, to the organism, and perhaps to the community and beyond. Here's one example: autophagy, a process in which a cell sequesters part of its contents to be self-digested and recycled, is mediated by the endocannabinoid system. While this process keeps normal cells alive, allowing them to maintain a balance between the synthesis, degradation, and subsequent recycling of cellular products, it has a deadly effect on malignant tumor cells, causing them to consume themselves in a programmed cellular suicide. The death of cancer cells, of course, promotes homeostasis and survival at the level of the entire organism.

Endocannabinoids and cannabinoids are also found at the intersection of the body's various systems, allowing communication and coordination between different cell types. At the site of an injury, for example, cannabinoids can be found decreasing the release of activators and sensitizers from the injured tissue, stabilizing the nerve cell to prevent excessive firing and pain signaling, and calming nearby immune cells to dampen the release of pro-inflammatory substances. Three different mechanisms of action on three different cell types for a single purpose: minimize the pain and damage caused by the injury.

The endocannabinoid system, with its complex actions in our immune system, nervous system, and all of the body's organs, is literally a bridge between body and mind.

The placebo effect, perhaps the greatest evidence that our internal pharmacy can match the effects of most medical treatments when properly stimulated by belief, is dependent on endocannabinoid activity. By understanding the ECS we begin to see a mechanism that explains how states of consciousness can promote health or disease.

In addition to regulating our internal and cellular homeostasis, cannabinoids influence a person's relationship with the external environment. Socially, the administration of cannabinoids clearly alters human behavior, often promoting sharing, humor, and creativity. By mediating neurogenesis (the growth of nerve cells), neuronal plasticity (the brain's ability to reorganize itself by forming new neural connections throughout life), and learning, cannabinoids may directly influence a person's open-mindedness and ability to move beyond limiting patterns of thought and behavior from past situations. Reformatting these old patterns is an essential part of health in our quickly changing environment.

What Are Cannabinoid Receptors?

All vertebrate species share the endocannabinoid system as an essential part of life and adaptation to environmental changes. Sea squirts and salamanders also have an ECS. By comparing the genetics of cannabinoid receptors in different species, scientists estimate that the endocannabinoid system evolved in primitive animals over 600 million years ago. In contrast, the plant cannabis evolved ~32 million years ago.

While it may seem we know a lot about cannabinoids, the twenty-four thousand scientific articles have just begun to shed light on the subject. Large gaps likely exist in our current understanding, and the complexity of interactions between various cannabinoids, cell types, systems and individual organisms challenges scientists to think about physiology and health in new ways. The following brief overview summarizes what we do know.

Cannabinoid receptors are present throughout the body, embedded in cell membranes, and are believed to be more numerous than any other receptor type in the body. Researchers have identified two cannabinoid receptors: CB1, predominantly present in the nervous system, connective tissues, gonads, glands, and organs; and CB2, predominantly found in the immune system and its associated structures. Many tissues contain both CB1 and CB2 receptors, each linked to a different action. When cannabinoid receptors are stimulated, a variety of physiologic processes ensue. Researchers speculate there may be a third cannabinoid receptor waiting to be discovered or named.

Endocannabinoids are the substances our bodies naturally make to stimulate these receptors. (Endo- is the Latin word meaning internal or within.) The two most well understood of these molecules are called anandamide and 2-arachidonoylglycerol (2-AG). They are synthesized on-demand from cell membrane arachidonic acid (omega-6) derivatives, have a local effect and short half-life before being degraded by the enzymes fatty acid amide hydrolase (FAAH) and monoacylglycerol lipase (MAGL).

Phytocannabinoids are plant substances that stimulate cannabinoid receptors. (Phyto- is the Latin word meaning related to plants.) Delta-9-tetrahydrocannabinol, or THC, is the most psychoactive and certainly the most famous of the phytocannabinoids, but other cannabinoids such as cannabidiol (CBD) and cannabinol (CBN) are gaining the interest of researchers due to a variety of healing properties. Most phytocannabinoids have been isolated from cannabis sativa, but other medical herbs, such as echinacea purpura (the well known purple coneflower plant), have been found to contain non-psychoactive cannabinoids as well.

Interestingly, the cannabis plant also uses the cannabinoids to promote its own health and prevent disease. Cannabinoids have antioxidant properties that protect the leaves and flowering structures from ultraviolet radiation - cannabinoids neutralize the harmful free radicals generated by UV rays, protecting the cells. In humans, free radicals cause aging, cancer, and impaired healing. Antioxidants found in plants have long been promoted as natural supplements to prevent free radical harm.

Laboratories can also produce cannabinoids. Synthetic THC, marketed as dronabinol (Marinol), and nabilone (Cesamet), a THC analog, are both FDA approved drugs for the treatment of severe nausea and wasting syndrome. Some clinicians and researchers have found them helpful in the off-label treatment of chronic pain, migraine, PTSD, and other conditions. Many other synthetic cannabinoids are used in animal research, and some have potency up to 600 times that of THC.

Cannabis, The Endocannabinoid System, And Good Health
As we continue to sort through the

emerging science of cannabis and cannabinoids, one thing remains clear: a functional cannabinoid system is essential for health. From embryonic implantation on the wall of our mother's uterus, to nursing and growth, to responding to injuries, endocannabinoids help us survive in a quickly changing and increasingly hostile environment. As I realized this, I began to wonder: can an individual enhance his/her cannabinoid system by taking supplemental cannabis? Beyond treating symptoms, beyond even curing disease, can cannabis help us prevent disease and promote health by stimulating an ancient system that is hard-wired into all of us?

I now believe the answer is yes. Research has shown that small doses of cannabinoids from cannabis can signal the body to make more endocannabinoids and build more cannabinoid receptors. This may be why many first-time cannabis users don't feel an effect, but by their second or third time using the herb they have built more cannabinoid receptors and are ready to respond. More receptors increase a person's sensitivity to cannabinoids; smaller doses have larger effects, and the individual has an enhanced baseline of endocannabinoid activity. I believe that small, regular doses of cannabis might act as a tonic to our most central physiologic healing system.

Other evidence suggests that very low doses of phytocannabinoids can protect the heart, brain, blood vessels, and other organs in the case of injury or disease.

Many physicians cringe at the thought of recommending a botanical substance and are outright mortified by the idea of smoking a medicine. Our medical system is more comfortable with single, isolated substances that can be swallowed or injected. Unfortunately, this model significantly limits the therapeutic potential of cannabinoids. Unlike synthetic derivatives, herbal cannabis may contain over one hundred different cannabinoids, including THC, which all work synergistically to produce better medical effects and less side effects than THC alone. While cannabis is safe and works well when smoked, many patients prefer to avoid respiratory irritation and instead use a vaporizer, cannabis tincture, or topical salve. Scientific inquiry and patient testimonials both indicate that herbal cannabis has superior medical qualities to synthetic cannabinoids.

In 1902 Thomas Edison said, "There were never so many able, active minds at work on the

MEDICAL CAN

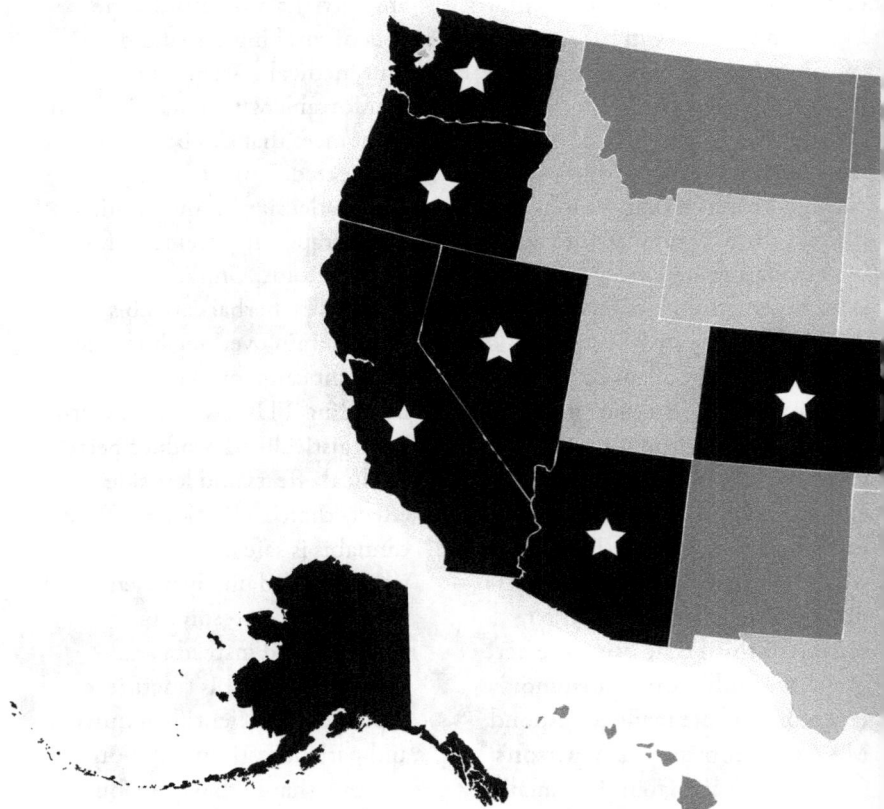

Med & Rec   **Med Only**   CBD O

NABIS LAWS

nly | None | ☆ Mary's Available

★ VT
NH
MA
RI
CT
NJ
DE
DC
★ MD

problems of disease as now, and all their discoveries are tending toward the simple truth that you can't improve on nature." Cannabinoid research has proven this statement is still valid.

So, is it possible that medical cannabis could be the most useful remedy to treat the widest variety of human diseases and conditions, a component of preventative healthcare, and an adaptive support in our increasingly toxic, carcinogenic environment? Yes. This was well known to the indigenous medical systems of ancient India, China, and Tibet, and is becoming increasingly well known by Western science. Of course, we need more human-based research studying the effectiveness of cannabis, but the evidence base is already large and growing constantly, despite the numerous federal obstacles to cannabis-related research.

Does your doctor understand the benefit of medical cannabis? Can he or she advise you in the proper indications, dosage, and route of administration? Likely not. Despite the two largest U.S. physician associations (American Medical Association and American College of Physicians) calling for more research, the U.S. Congress prohibiting federal interference in states' medical cannabis programs, a 5,000 year

history of safe therapeutic use, and a huge amount of published research, most doctors know little or nothing about medical cannabis. This is changing, in part because the public is demanding it. People want safe, natural and inexpensive treatments that stimulate our bodies' ability to self-heal and help our population improve its quality of life. Medical cannabis is one such solution. 🌿

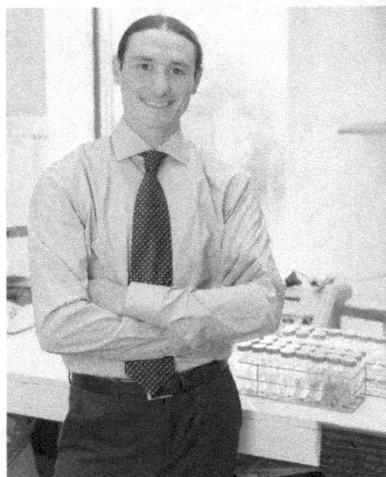

Dr. Dustin Sulak is an integrative medicine physician with an emphasis in osteopathy, energy medicine, mind-body medicine, and medical cannabis. His clinical practice focuses on treating refractory conditions in adults and children with an individualized, health-centered approach. Dr. Sulak is the founder of Integr8 Health, a medical practice with 3 locations in New England that treat over 18,000 patients with medical cannabis, Tested Labs, a cannabis analytic laboratory, and Healer.com, an medical cannabis education resource.

HERE'S THE THING: A MOTHER'S STORY

By: Heather Jackson
CEO, The Realm of Caring

Here's the thing about pharmaceuticals. Many of them often operate via the same mechanism of action. They are frequently just repackaged with a shiny bow, high price tag, and a new name which is difficult to pronounce. There's a problem with targeting the same mechanism; especially when it comes to my son who has a catastrophic epilepsy diagnosis, or for anyone dealing with a chronic health condition taking pharmaceuticals that are not helping. If the particular mechanism of action doesn't work to stop your symptoms or the disease, then the next four drugs that operate on the same mechanism probably won't work either. This was our personal experience. My son Zaki went through seventeen pharmaceuticals, most with similar, often identical ways they worked in the body. None of them actually stopped his seizures and all came with a laundry list of side effects like lethargy, blindness and even death, to name a few.

As a parent whose sole purpose is to protect their child, I could not just give up. Nor was it a good choice to recycle back through drugs which didn't work. I knew I needed to keep researching.

I began to consider cannabis in late 2011 after my son's EEG (electroencephalogram) showed seizure activity every 10 seconds, and he was receiving hospice palliative services.

Here's the thing about educating yourself. It is empowering. I began to research how cannabis works in the body. Cannabidiol (CBD) is one of many cannabinoids found in cannabis and hemp. When discussing CBD research, I have heard doctors say it is "messy" to study. Well, I can understand their opinion because it does almost fifty different things in our body. 50! That doesn't even take into consideration the other almost 400 natural chemical components of the plant. Doctors are accustomed to an isolated chemical that goes in and does one thing they may or may not be able to measure. What may be viewed as "messy" to them, made me rub my hands together with excitement! I was finally going to have the option to try something new for my son whose brain could not take a rest from the electrical shocks coming like clockwork.

Here's the thing about the endocannabinoid system (ECS). I do not have initials behind my name. I am not a doctor, I am "just a mom." But neither I nor you need to be a neuroscientist to learn and discover this unique system in our body. In fact, it is the largest regulating system in our body. It is responsible for bringing the body into balance which is called Homeostasis. Let that roll off of your tongue a couple of times. When is the last time you went to your doctor and he or she said, "Let me see how we can get you back in homeostasis?" Our bodies are meant to heal themselves. This idea sounded pretty great to me after almost a decade of trying to keep my boy alive. Healing sounded like bliss, an unattainable utopian idea. Trying something that worked like nothing else we had tried previously sounded like the next place to start. Boy am I glad we did. He is now approaching 4 years seizure free, we got to meet our boy for the first time, and his brain is healing with the aid of a little plant on a phenomenal regulation system.

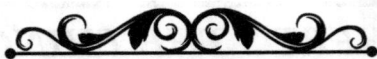

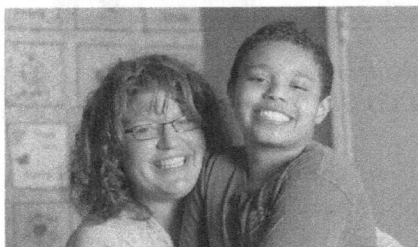

Heather Jackson is the CEO of the Realm of Caring Foundation. Her passion for medical cannabis came after her son Zaki displayed complete seizure remission on Charlotte's Web Hemp Oil in 2012. She went from caring for Zaki while he received hospice palliative services to helping families from all over the world educate themselves and access this therapy.

She has now dedicated her life to furthering research, education and advocacy into this often misunderstood therapy option. The Realm of Caring has experienced explosive growth from tracking their original few children to engaging over 6,000 in research protocols in two years with over 25,000 members and no slowing down in sight. The Realm of Caring has the largest IRB approved registry in the world, and is currently tracking the largest population using cannabinoids for epilepsy. The Realm of Caring has received both national and international attention and has been featured on CNN with Sanjay Gupta, Dateline, The View, New York Times, National Geographic, 60 minutes and many more.

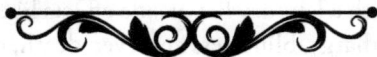

HOW TO FIND IT:
SEARCHING FOR MEDICAL CANNABIS INFORMATION

By Alice O'Leary-Randall
Executive Editor,
Mary's Cannabis Primer

An important element of becoming a medical cannabis patient (or a caregiver to a medical cannabis patient) is the willingness to continually learn. Using cannabis medically is not as simple as "Take this pill, once a day." To use cannabis successfully you must become an advocate for your own health and learn all that you can about this plant. Why? Because every day brings a better understanding of cannabis and how it helps our physiologic and mental health. Remember, the endogenous cannabinoid system (ECS) was only discovered in 1992. Once researchers began to understand the true significance of the ECS there was an explosion of research that is still ongoing. This means not only are scientists discovering more about the workings of the ECS but they are also developing new delivery forms (i.e., transdermal patches, pills, tinctures, etc.) This will translate into better ways of treating some of mankind's most intractable diseases.

So, I know that some of you are probably saying, "Well, I don't want to study. I want to get well." Of course you do. But it is important to remember that no one cares as much about you as you. No one. Not your doctors or your family. It is up to you and if you are reading this publication you have demonstrated that you want to be in charge of your medical care. You've already taken the biggest step.

Fortunately there are many tools available to individuals seeking information about medical cannabis and the ECS. The first is the internet. In fact, there is almost too much information on the internet. You need to have a plan when you begin using the internet for more than just restaurant reviews and movie tickets.

You might want to start with basic, disease-specific websites, many of which are hosted by non-profit associations. Remember that these serve a wide-array of clients so the language can be bland and often noncommittal. In others, the website may not endorse the medical use of cannabis, just the

57

opposite. But these websites can help educate us on the basics of whichever disease we are researching. They can become an excellent source of fundamental information.

There are also some very good websites that specialize in medical cannabis information at every level of understanding from beginner to the seasoned activist. Explore as many as you have the time for. Simply type "medical cannabis" in your browser and take your pick.

Be sure to make use of your browser's Bookmark feature. Bookmarks provide a means of organizing our information into folders, just as we have done for years with those manila, tab-cut folders that went into the file drawers. Web bookmarks are the equivalent of this. When you see an article you want to retain you click Bookmarks in the menu and then select which folder to add it to. There is no right or wrong way to name folders so don't get hung up on that. Organize it so that you will know where to go to find the information later.

Once you have become acquainted with the specifics of your disease you may then want to start looking for scientific articles. Now, some of these articles can be really technical and, frankly, unreadable by the lay person. Most scientific articles, however,

have what is called an "Abstract" that will briefly describe the research and the conclusion. For most people this is all you need to read. You will also find that printing out a copy of the Abstract and giving it to your healthcare professionals may help educate them too.

By the way, consider using Google Scholar when you start looking for more detailed scientific research. Google Scholar limits its search to scientific journals, government documents and the like. There are no advertisements but be advised that many sites will charge you to read the full article. However, as mentioned above, the Abstract will normally give you the full story and it is displayed free of charge.

Make your search as specific as you can and include your disease category. For example, search for "glaucoma and medical cannabis." Cannabis is the preferred term to use and most scientific articles will use this proper botanical term. But it is also interesting to do a search for "glaucoma and medical marijuana," just to see the difference in what appears.

Learning as much as we can about the medicines that we use is good practice whether the drug is a conventional prescription or medical cannabis. As Heather Davis notes in her article "Here's The Thing," (page 19) education is "empowering". There will be no tests. You don't need to be an expert about cannabis but you do need to become an expert about you.

Simply by starting the process you have passed the real test. Failure lies in not learning about this fascinating medication that has helped mankind for millennia. 🌿

NOTES: _____

In March 2018, Heather Jackson reported that her son, Zaki, is continuing to do well. He has mild, infrequent seizures which Heather feels may be related to the onset of puberty. She has tried other cannabinoids (THC, THCA, CBN, CBC) but none have been as effective as CBD. Heather continues to work as executive director of the Realm of Caring in Colorado Springs.

As of April 2018, Mary's Medicinals products are available in Arizona, Colorado, California, Florida, Illinois, Maryland, Nevada, Oregon, Vermont and Washington.

Mary's

CANNABIS PRIMER

issue #4

CANNABIS & NUTRITION

The Incredibly Versatile Cannabis Plant
A Dietician's Perspective on Cannabis
Nutrition and Cannabis
Healthy! Nutritional Value of Hemp Seeds
Cannabis and a Healthy Lifestyle
Sam Skipper and the Nutritional Power of Cannabis
Hemp or Cannabis? Which is More Nutritional?
Cannabis Nutrition Resources

EDITOR'S NOTE

Cannabis and Nutrition

The first time I considered cannabis as a nutritional substance was in the early 1990s. The AIDS epidemic was in its fury and people with AIDS (PWAs) were desperate for anything that could alleviate their suffering. I was working with my late husband, Robert C. Randall, at the Alliance for Cannabis Therapeutics and we were hearing from more and more PWAs about their use of cannabis. Some, like Sam Skipper, were getting arrested. Sam told Bob that he would "graze" his way through his cannabis plants which was the first time either of us had heard about eating the raw plant. Sam must have been doing something right because he is still alive, nearly thirty years later.

Sam was following his instincts, just as millions of humans have since the beginning of time. Cannabis is ancient and so is the system within us that is designed to receive cannabinoid-like substances. The endogenous cannabinoid system (ECS) was only discovered in the early 1990s, around the time that Sam Skipper was diagnosed with AIDS and began to piece together the importance of cannabis in his own life. It was relatively simple: when Sam used cannabis his T-cells, those markers of the body's ability to fight infection, would go up. When Sam didn't have cannabis his T-cells collapsed. Over and over again we were hearing from AIDS patients who told us the same thing: cannabis was keeping them alive. Sam's story is covered in the excerpt from our book, *Marijuana Rx: The Patients' Fight for Medicinal Pot* which can be found on page 16.

Today we are beginning to understand just how important the ECS actually is to our health and well being. Like many others, I have become convinced that cannabis could well become a nutritional supplement in the future. Already people are using CBD (the dramatic cannabis component that has proven so useful to children with intractable epilepsy) as a daily supplement to help maintain their homeostasis (physiological balance). This issue of *The Primer* takes a look at the use and benefits of cannabis as a nutritional supplement with several articles from the internet (thanks to Leafly.com and cannabis.info.com for permission to print) and a couple of original articles by Dr. Joe Cohen of Holos Health (page 14) and Marla Perez of Mary's Medicinals (page 6).

Justin Kander returns to *The Primer* (see Issue 2, Cancer and Cannabis) with his usual insightfulness (page 10). Justin provides a list of available supplements that will help our ECS work more efficiently. He reminds us that "The more you do to support your ECS, the more your ECS will support you." Advice for the ages.

Alice O'Leary-Randall
Editor in Chief - Mary's Cannabis Primer
alice@marysmedicinals.com
www.aliceolearyrandall.com

THE INCREDIBLY VERSATILE CANNABIS PLANT

By Marla Perez,
Account Executive, Mary's Medicinals

The versatility of the cannabis plant yields a wide range of use. Not only does it have deep medicinal and healing properties to treat symptoms of chronic disease, it also has properties that can be used recreationally. Our culture seems so fixated on the idea that cannabis is used only for the chronically ill or for those that are seeking the recreational psychoactive high, that it tends to miss the people who fall in between. One component of the plant that is overlooked is its potential ability to be used interdependently with the elements that contribute to a greater quality of life including physical fitness, sleep and a nutrient dense diet.

Sleep

Quality sleep is an integral part of a healthy lifestyle as its been shown to play a critical role in immune function, metabolism, and other vital functions. Scientists have gone to great lengths to study the role of sleep on our body and multiple studies have shown insufficient sleep to be directly correlated to heart disease, mood disorders, obesity, and diabetes. Cannabinol (CBN), a cannabinoid that results from the degradation of tetrahydrocannabinol (THC), has deep relaxing properties that offers sleep support by allowing your body to fall into a deeper and more restful stage of sleep, known as the REM (rapid eye movement) stage, relaxing not only your body, but also your mind.

Physical Fitness

Exercise has recently taken center stage as being a major component to maintaining health but the reality is that it's no easy task. During strenuous exercise, our bodies work overtime to deliver enough oxygen to our working muscles as aerobic (with oxygen) methods are the most efficient way to deliver energy to our system. However, when oxygen supply is insufficient and energy is needed faster than we can produce, glucose is broken down and metabolized anaerobically (without oxygen) into pyruvate which in turn converts to a substance called lactate, also known as lactic acid. Lactic acid accumulation results in an increase in acidity in muscle cells causing the burn associated with exercise and also inflammation as the muscle begins to break down. Although this sounds counterproductive, it's a natural defense mechanism to prevent further damage and furthermore, provides an opportunity for our body to rebuild and recover itself coming back much stronger. Cannabidiol (CBD) and tetrahydrocannabinol (THC) have known analgesic and anti-inflammatory properties which can provide support for long term, sustained muscular recovery and growth. As research continues to offer evidence of different properties that other cannabinoid profiles offer, we can expand the use of cannabis for any fitness regimen e.g. cannabichromene (CBC) which has bone growth promoting properties, for joint support during high impact exercises.

Nutrition

The obesity epidemic is well documented. It's the result of an over-fed and under-active population. As research continues to head in the direction of what it means to maintain healthy eating habits, more evidence is starting to point towards plant-based diets. More organic options are becoming available, and holistic options are more preferred. Studies show that specific cannabinoid properties potentially offer the same regulatory functions as vitamins and minerals do and are beneficial not only to treat symptoms of chronic disease, but also as a preventative measure through proactive endocannabinoid therapy. Essentially, we can shift the collective perspective of the cannabis plant as a "drug", and view cannabinoids of the cannabis plant to be analogous to the vitamins and minerals of fruits and vegetables. Although maintaining a healthy lifestyle is a result of individual choices, cannabis offers a multitude of various properties that can be used to support healthier habits to increase the quality of life. As we continue to develop our knowledge of the various properties of the 80+ known cannabinoids, it's important to consider the various implications of its uses to bridge the gap between sickness and health. 🍎

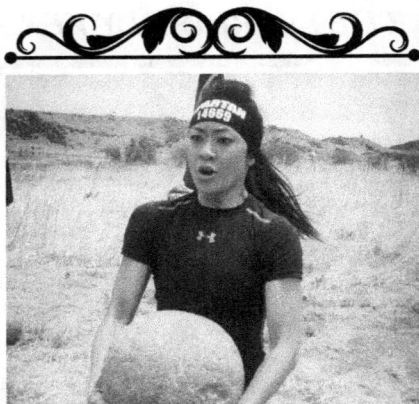

Marla Perez is a passionate individual who believes in the importance of holistic health for mind body and soul. As a former personal trainer and health coach of seven years, she has created a foundation of knowledge utilizing several techniques such as metabolic conditioning, nutritional programming, fitness designing, hormonal balancing and DNA testing. Now working as an Account Executive for Mary's Medicinals in Northern Colorado, she looks forward to educating and offering the public an alternative and holistic form of Medicine.

A DIETITIAN'S PERSPECTIVE ON CANNABIS

By Jessica Aragona

Reproduced with permission of Leafly.com

https://www.leafly.com/news/health/a-dietitians-perspective-on-cannabis

Cannabis can save the world. A bold statement perhaps, but potentially true nonetheless. As a dietitian, when I look at the cannabis plant, I first see its nutritional value as a vegetable, loaded with vitamins, minerals, and antioxidants. I also know that essentially cannabis is hemp, and hemp hits a home run every time when it comes to nutritional value (among its other thousands of industrial uses).

A quick nutritional summary of hemp:

- Great source of complete protein
- 100% vegan
- Dairy-free
- Gluten-free
- Easy to digest
- High in healthy Omega-3 and Omega-6 fatty acids

Wow — what a power house!

As a holistic healthcare professional, I recognize and highly respect the diversity of cannabis in its uses as a medicine to heal and repair both the body and the mind. It is my opinion that cannabis may not only be the best medicine, but also the most nutritious plant known to humankind thus far.

The Nutritional Health Benefits of Raw Cannabis

While the exact nutritional profile of cannabis has yet to be determined, it seems safe to assume that the cannabis plant, including the seeds, is most likely just as nutritious as hemp, if not more so.

What's being discovered now is the nutritional power and overall beneficial health effects of raw cannabis. Raw cannabis is not psychoactive unless heated, and it contains powerful disease-fighting compounds known as cannabinoids. Of these compounds, the most frequently studied are Tetrahydrocannabinol (THC) and Cannabidiol (CBD).

When used just as you would any other vegetable (in a smoothie, salad, sauté, juiced), cannabis appears to provide some pretty awesome health benefits. You may have heard of Kristen Peskuski-Courtney, a woman who struggled with multiple chronic illnesses which left her all but debilitated. After years of pharmaceutical intervention to no avail, her health dramatically improved through the power of raw cannabis juicing. The man behind this method of ingestion is Dr. William Courtney, a medical doctor and huge promoter of the "raw greens" cannabis movement.

From Dr. Courtney:

"Whether Sativa, Indica, Ruderalis, male, female, hermaphrodite, native, feral, bred for fiber, seeds or medicinal resin, cannabis is the best source for [beneficial cannabinoids]...Over 50 patients have used only [cannabinoids] to put their cancer in remission; and over 150 have found symptomatic relief."

What does that tell you? What it says to me is that there is some powerful research being done and treatment methods being delivered out there to very sick patients, and they are all based on raw cannabis.

Dr. Courtney has researched the benefits of raw cannabis and has come to the following conclusions:

- Smoking cannabis may not treat the disease, only the symptoms
- Therapeutic levels of cannabinoids are better achieved through ingestion
- When cannabis is heated or burned, the chemical structure of the plant compounds are changed, specifically the acidity of THC, which alters its ability to be therapeutic
- Raw cannabis activates the brain's cannabinoid system, which triggers antioxidants
- These antioxidants act as a "cleaner" and remove damaged cells from the body
- Raw cannabis improves the efficiency of the cells in our body
- Creating oils, butters or eating the raw plant is the best way to get the necessary beneficial compounds

Looking to incorporate more "green" into your daily diet? If you're interested in exploring the benefits of raw cannabis, here are some tips and recommendations:

- Raw cannabis can be used every day, multiple times a day by anyone of any age.
- Raw cannabis is not psychoactive unless it is heated, meaning there are no worries of mental or physical impairment after consuming
- Raw cannabis can be added to smoothies, juices, and salads
- Like any other herb or seasoning, ground up raw buds can be sprinkled on top of soups, stews, oatmeal, yogurt, or pudding
- Juicing specifically takes a lot of material; Dr. Courtney suggests 20-30 big shade leaves or 2-3 raw buds (2-3 inches in length) per day for therapeutic benefits
- Having your own garden at home is helpful as access to this quantity of raw product may be difficult or illegal in your state. 🌿

....

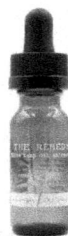

Mary's Nutritionals
Remedy Oil
Available for delivery to all 50 states at
marysnutritionals.com

....

NUTRITION AND CANNABIS

By Justin Kander,
Research & Development Coordinator,
Aunt Zelda's

The optimal use of medical cannabis goes far beyond consumption of the plant. While dosing, cultivar selection, and THC:CBD ratios are important, all of this can mean little if other health factors are not addressed. The most important contributor to our health is arguably nutrition. Everything we put into our bodies ultimately becomes us, so if our raw fuel is without substance, our cells will not function properly. Furthermore, in the context of cannabis medicine, our endocannabinoid systems (ECS) are likely impaired by poor nutrition, which limits the efficacy of cannabis. On the other hand, with the right nutrition, we can prime our endocannabinoid systems to benefit as much as possible from any cannabinoid therapy.

Priming the ECS

The standard American diet is tremendously unbalanced, with most people consuming far more omega-6 fatty acids. While omega-6 is still important, having too much can contribute to chronic inflammation in the body, which may contribute to a wide variety of diseases, including autoimmune disorders and cancer. Foods rich in omega-3s, like fish, eggs, walnuts, and hemp seed, can help to balance the omega-6 to omega-3 ratio.

A 2011 study in Nature Neuroscience found that mice with omega-3 deficiency experienced impaired CB1 receptor functioning (https://www.ncbi.nlm.nih.gov/pubmed/21278728). The receptors became disconnected from the second messengers which relay their signals of activation. This phenomenon was shown to have a measurable, adverse effect in mice, impairing their emotional behavior. While more research is needed, it is quite possible that omega-3 deficiency and associated impaired cannabinoid receptor signaling is an underlying factor contributing to widespread anxiety and depression.

Much scientific interest has emerged in recent years surrounding the gut microbiome, the collection of bacteria residing in the gastrointestinal tract. Some research suggests microbiome imbalances may contribute to the formation of inflammatory bowel disease, diabetes, and other systemic conditions (https://www.ncbi.nlm.nih.gov/pubmed/26770121). Probiotic supplements and foods are now being used to treat some of these conditions. Among the many benefits of probiotics, they appear to work in part through the ECS. One of the most well-studied probiotic strains, Lactobacillus acidophilus, has been shown to upregulate CB2 receptors on human intestinal cells (https://www.ncbi.nlm.nih.gov/pubmed/17159985). Interestingly, the bacteria then appear to induce painkilling effects through activation of the CB2 receptors. Chronic inflammation is another significant contributor to disease. The ECS has an anti-inflammatory function (https://www.ncbi.nlm.nih.gov/pubmed/24529123), and it is possible that chronic inflammation leads to a depletion of endocannabinoids or excessive taxation on the receptors. Therefore, it makes sense to consume meals rich in anti-inflammatory foods and low in pro-inflammatory foods. The Mediterranean diet is a great starting point for a delicious, effective anti-inflammatory diet. Fish, eggs, fruits, vegetables, nuts, and seeds, along with olive oil and red wine, embody the Mediterranean diet. Most seasoning herbs have anti-inflammatory activity, with some of the strongest being ginger, turmeric, and basil.

Activation of the cannabinoid receptors is one of the major ways cannabis acts medicinally. Using nutritional strategies to upregulate the receptors and enhance their function can make cannabis work better. This means that a smaller amount can be used to achieve the same therapeutic effect, or an overall higher level of healing can be reached. The more you do to support your ECS, the more your ECS will support you. 🌿

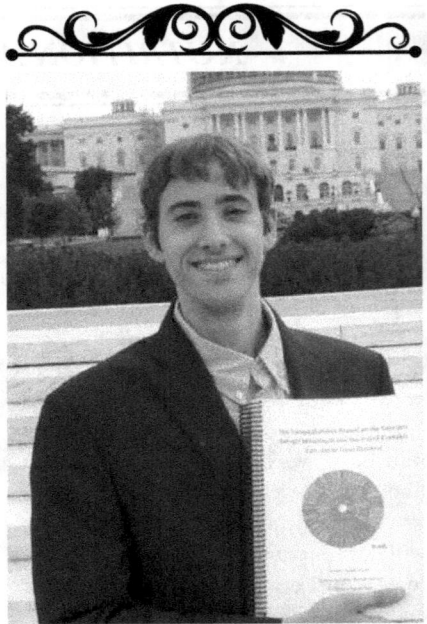

Justin Kander has been an activist for the use of cannabis extract medicine since 2008. He has written several books on cannabis medicine including *The Comprehensive Report on the Cannabis Extract Movement and Enhancing Your Endocannabinoid System*, Kander has presented at medical cannabis conferences in Australia, Costa Rica, and the United States. He now works as the Research and Development Coordinator for Aunt Zelda's, where he writes educational material and helps produce cannabis extracts for seriously ill patients in the state of California.

HEALTHY! NUTRITIONAL VALUE OF HEMP SEEDS

By Cannabis.info
Used With Permission

https://www.cannabis.info/en/healthy-nutritional-value-hemp-seeds

Bring up the topic of hemp seeds at your next social gathering and you're likely to turn a few heads. The sheer mention of anything related to cannabis is a lot for some people to handle, immediately conjuring up a mental image of getting high. In actuality, consuming hemp seeds does not result in any psychotropic effects. However, they do provide a myriad of nutritional benefits like no other seed on earth.

The verdict? Hemp is healthy! Nutritional value of hemp seeds cannot be overstated, as they feature a complex profile of proteins, fats, vitamins and minerals, that reduce and prevent life threatening diseases, such as cancer and heart disease.

Rich Source Of Protein

Hemp seeds are an excellent source of protein. Containing all 9 essential amino acids (EAA's), that the human body does not produce, hemp seeds are second only to soybeans in protein content. In total, hemp seeds contain all 20 amino acids known to man, helping to stimulate muscle growth and strengthen the body's natural defense system.

For vegetarians and vegans, hemp seeds are a perfectly valid meat substitute at around 10g of protein per three tablespoons. Seeds are relatively high in calories as well, making them a perfect dietary addition for athletes and other highly active individuals.

Excellent Source Of Fats

Some of the most important nutritional implications of hemp seeds originate in its rich concentration of fats. Indeed, over 30% of hemp seeds are made up of fats, with an uneven split of 75-80% polyunsaturated fats and 9-11% saturated fats. As such, hemp seeds are "perfectly balanced" with a 3:1 ratio of omega-6 to omega-3 fatty acids. Humans need both types of these fats to be healthy. Contrary to popular belief, some types of fats are good for you!

Hemp contains a naturally occurring compound known as gamma linolenic acid or GLA. GLA is categorized as an omega-6 fatty acid, that shows particular promise in the realm of cancer treatments and promotes many other health benefits as well.

Heart And Hormone Health

GLA is also essential in maintaining proper cardiovascular and hormonal health. The omega-3 fatty acids help to reduce inflammation and ease pain. Hemp seeds contain arginine, an amino acid, that produces nitric acid, which ultimately helps to reduce your risk of heart disease. Hemp seeds are quickly being recognized as beneficial for premenstrual syndrome (PMS). GLA produces prostaglandin E1 to reduce the adverse effects of the hormone prolactin, which is responsible for causing symptoms of pain. GLA can help to ease the physical and emotional symptoms that many women experience.

Good For Digestive Health

Hemp seeds contain both soluble and insoluble fibers, that encourage healthy bowel movements and overall digestive health. By cultivating a healthy digestive system, these fibers help manage symptoms of high cholesterol and strengthen probiotics for total immune health.

High Doses Of Vitamins And Minerals

A wealth of phytonutrients are contained in hemp seeds, making these the ideal avenue for receiving your necessary vitamins and minerals. Among some of the most occurring minerals are calcium, iron, phosphorus and zinc. Vitamins run the gamut with at least seven appearing in different concentrations, including vitamin A and vitamin B12. This strong phytocomplex allows for consumers to ingest a well-rounded course of nutrients, without having to purchase many different supplements contained in capsules and tinctures.

Skin Relief

Hemp seeds contain antioxidants, that penetrate deep into the skin to relieve inflammation, dryness and redness. Hemp seed oil can be found in many popular skincare and haircare products, that spur healthy cell growth. Hemp oils frequently appear as ingredients in eczema treatments, moisturizers and can be applied to help prevent acne. Hemp seeds encourage a quicker recovery from superficial wounds as the superfood does its best to supplement natural skin and cell regeneration.

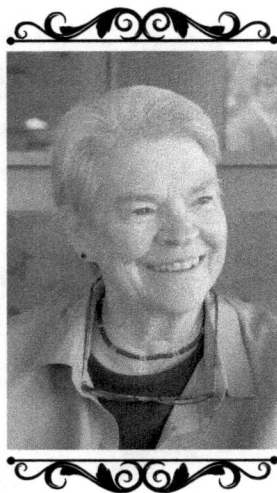

Primer's editor-in-chief, Alice O'Leary-Randall, is a true medical cannabis pioneer with more than forty years in the issue. To learn more about Alice please visit: **aliceolearyrandall.com**

Non-Psychoactive

Before moving any further, it's necessary to squash the rumor, that ingesting hemp seeds will make you feel high. You can rest assured this is not the case. While it's true, that hemp is a genetic of the cannabis sativa plant, it contains negligible levels of THC. You will never have to worry about getting hit with a major stone half an hour after sprinkling some hemp seeds on your lunch. Years of stringent regulations have made consumers feel, that anything associated with cannabis is bad and unhealthy when in reality, the opposite is true!

Cooking With Hemp Seeds

Surprisingly, hemp seeds aren't actually seeds at all – they're nuts. Once you taste them, it will all make sense. The beauty of this product is, that it can be infused into so many different types of food and beverage. If you're short on time, you can easily sprinkle hemp seeds over hot dishes and salads. At the same time, you can blend them into smoothies and shakes to add an all-natural protein supplement to your regular routine.

Anywhere you'd put chia seeds, you can easily sub in hemp.

Since hemp seeds are hunger suppressants, they naturally facilitate weight loss. Eating them as a snack in the form of a energy bar is a great way to get good fats and protein on the go, without having to craft an entire meal. This is especially useful for those with busy jobs who eat their lunch with one hand and type with the other.

How Amazing Is Hemp?!

It isn't outrageous to deem hemp a miracle plant. In addition to containing game-changing cannabinoids like THC and CBD, as well as aromatic terpenes, hemp also provides a well rounded course of nutritional benefits, that inspires real impacts on human emotional and physical health.

Hemp is healthy! Nutritional value of hemp seeds cannot be overstated, as they feature a complex profile of proteins, fats, vitamins and minerals, that reduce and prevent life threatening diseases. 🌿

CANNABIS AND A HEALTHY LIFESTYLE

By Joseph Cohen, D.O.
Holos Health, Boulder, CO

"The ultimate adaptogenic herb" is an apt description of cannabis. We've evolved this amazing endocannabinoid system (ECS) with receptors in our brain, immune system and throughout our body. Intricate and complex, the primary function of our ECS is to provide us with balance and homeostasis--both physical and emotional. The cannabis plant produces phytocannabinoids with the same chemical structure as our endocannabinoids. They have the ability to bind to these receptors and, together with terpenes, create an entourage effect. In other words, we are wired for this plant! By helping us adapt to both internal and external forces, cannabis can do what no other plant or medicine can.

We cannot separate our physical and emotional self. Let's consider how cannabis can connect the emotional to the physical.

When we feel stressed, our brain sends signals to our adrenal glands, our flight or fight organs, that try to help us adapt to stress. Unfortunately, in these stressful times, our adrenals are having a difficult time handling so many stressors and, as a result, become fatigued, losing their ability to provide us with homeostasis. In addition to many other functions, our adrenals also play a vital role in hormone production and balance. When attacked by stress our neuroendocrine system may become dysfunctional therefore creating many challenges to our physical and emotional wellbeing.

THC and CBD are both known to have positive effects on reducing stress. THC helps us live in the now and not focus on yesterday and tomorrow. CBD is an excellent anti-anxiety drug and mitigates some of the untoward effects of THC. THC and CBD are the Yin-Yang of the plant, complementing one another. With the appropriate use of cannabis, we can decrease stressors and, therefore, both shed and prevent chronic disease.

Medicating with cannabis prior to exercise can have multiple benefits. When used correctly, cannabinoids can open our airways, therefore allowing greater flow of oxygen to our tissues. Many people report that their workout routine is more productive and enjoyable. Many people report that they are be able to incorporate meditation into their workout routine. Starting your day by micro-dosing with a short acting form of cannabis can assist you in reducing stress as well as encouraging positive behavior. 🌿

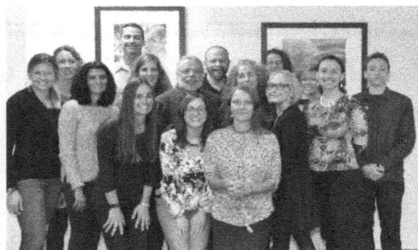

Dr. Cohen and staff of Holos Health

Dr. Cohen completed his residency training in 1979. He practiced in CT and CO before venturing to Wyoming to assist women of the Shoshoni and Arapaho tribes and to New Zealand where he worked with Maori women and families. After returning from New Zealand in 2009 Dr. Cohen ventured into the practice of cannabis medicine. Holos Health and Journey2Life were conceived in order to combine cannabis and functional medicine. In addition to studying cannabis extensively, Dr. Cohen feels that he learns more from patients than he does from reading medical cannabis textbooks and studies. He is currently authoring "The Cannabis Friendly Guide to Cannabis" and is teaching budtender training classes while maintaining a full-time medical practice in both Boulder and Denver.

By Robert C. Randall

An account of the first medical necessity trial in the state of California excerpted from Marijuana Rx: The Patients' Fight for Medicinal Pot

From Chapter 36

October 1993

Sam Skipper was arrested for growing marijuana in his home. I was contacted by his public defender, Juliana Humphrey.

Sam, 39, was a gay gardener who had watched 51 friends and lovers die from AIDS. First arrested for marijuana cultivation in 1990, Sam pled guilty because his lover was dying and he didn't want to cope with legal procedures. He was released on probation. Then, in March 1993, vice cops again raided Sam's modest suburban home and found 70 marijuana plants. Facing prison and death, Sam Skipper decided to fight.

After the vice cops collected evidence and left, Sam planted new seeds, then set off to a head shop in Oceanside where he found, and bought, the store's last copy of Marijuana & AIDS: Pot, Politics & PWAs in America, which Alice had published in late 1991. "It was such a pretty color," Sam said.

Sam's story was familiar. He had been HIV-positive for at least 4 years. His 51 friends who faithfully followed doctors' orders and took scores of toxic prescriptive potions were now all stone-cold dead. Sam looked great: healthy, high-spirited, well-nourished with good color. Why?

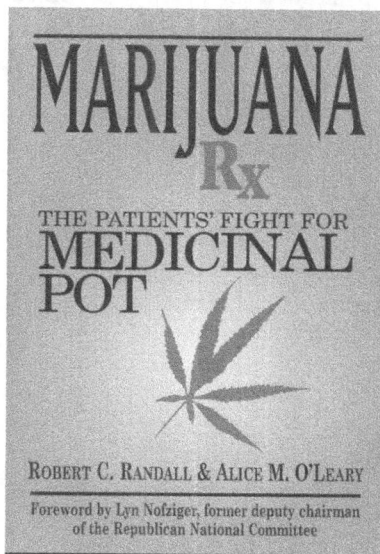

"Pot's kept me alive," Sam said without a trace of hesitation. Sam used marijuana in a different way than most AIDS patients. He would literally graze his way through his marijuana garden, pinching buds and munching on fresh leaves. He also mixed finely ground pot into peanut butter balls. Of modest height, he was a slightly pudgy 153 lbs.

Sam knew what it was like to slip off the tightrope. On the several occasions when he had no marijuana he lost 2 pounds a day.

Juliana Humphrey once saw Sam when he was without marijuana; pale, rail-thin, nauseated, unable to eat. Like Sam, Juliana had watched good friends with AIDS vanish. She was a deeply committed advocate.

In pre-trial motions I testified at length about my medical use of marijuana and that of AIDS patients like Kenny, Barbra, and Steve L.

As we moved on to the task of empaneling a jury I witnessed an awesome demonstration of how pervasive the acceptance of medical marijuana was in the general populace. Fourteen potential jurors—one after the other—took the stand and bluntly told the prosecutor there was no way they would convict a man with AIDS for the crime of medically employing marijuana. No way!

Sam Skipper's case dominated the San Diego news. A telephone poll conducted by one local TV station found 76% of the good citizens of conservative San Diego believed Sam Skipper had a right to medically use marijuana.

Not surprisingly, the jury acquitted him on all charges. ❧

*Excerpted from Marijuana Rx: The Patients' Fight for Medicinal Pot by Robert C. Randall and Alice M. O'Leary, © 1998. Published by Thunder's Mouth Press, New York, NY. Used with permission. Edited for space constraints.

HEMP OR CANNABIS? WHICH IS MORE NUTRITIONAL?

An ongoing source of confusion is the difference between hemp and cannabis. The short answer is: very little. Think of them as first cousins. By definition hemp has less tetrahydrocannabinoid than cannabis which is why it doesn't have the same psychoactive properties as cannabis. And hemp is predominantly used for industrial manufacturing — things like rope, paper, and fabric.

But today's hemp farmers are also breeding hemp plants that have high CBD percentages which has made hemp a good source for CBD oil. Many companies, including Mary's Nutritionals, use high-grade hemp for their CBD products.

Both hemp and cannabis provide excellent nutritional value.

Sam Skipper continues to live in the San Diego area following his acquittal. As of 2010 he was still alive and using cannabis, seventeen years after his trial for cultivation.

GLOSSARY

Adaptogenic - refers to the pharmacological concept whereby administration results in stabilization of physiological processes and promotion of homeostasis, for example, decreased cellular sensitivity to stress. Adaptogens not only increase the resistance to the adverse effects of long-term stress, the majority are also a tonic, immune-stimulating and increase general sense of well-being.

Allopathic - a system of medical practice that aims to combat disease by use of remedies (as drugs or surgery) producing effects different from or incompatible with those produced by the disease being treated.

Anandamide - a naturally occurring molecule which acts as a neurotransmitter, and which has a structure very similar to that of tetrahydrocannabinol, the active constituent of cannabis. It is a messenger molecule that plays a role in many bodily activities, including appetite, memory, pain, depression, and fertility - hence its name, which is derived from the word 'ananda' which means 'extreme delight' or 'bliss' in the Sanskrit language. Anandamide's discovery may lead to the development of an entirely new family of therapeutic drugs.

Angiogenesis - the physiological process through which new blood vessels form from pre-existing vessels. Angiogenesis is a normal and vital process in growth and development, as well as in wound healing and in the formation of granulation tissue. However, it is also a fundamental step in the transition of tumors from a benign state to a malignant one, leading to the use of angiogenesis inhibitors in the treatment of cancer. Some cannabinoids can inhibit angiogenesis.

Apoptosis - the death of cells that occurs as a normal and controlled part of an organism's growth or development.

CB1 and CB2 receptors - there are currently two known subtypes of cannabinoid receptors, termed CB1 and CB2. The CB1 receptor is expressed mainly in the brain (central nervous system or "CNS"), but also in the lungs, liver and kidneys. The CB2 receptor is expressed mainly in the immune system and in hematopoietic (blood production) cells.

CBD - cannabidiol, one of the principal components of the cannabis plant. CBD has demonstrated remarkable therapeutic properties especially in the treatment of intractable pediatric epilepsy.

Cultivars - an organism and especially one of an agricultural or horticultural variety or strain originating and persistent under cultivation.

Delta-9 THC - the primary psychoactive ingredient in cannabis. Delta-9 THC occurs when the naturally occurring THCA is heated either by smoking or through chemical procedures.

Decarboxylation - a chemical reaction that eliminates a carboxylic acid group from an organic compound. With respect to cannabis, decarboxylation occurs when the plant substance is heated, either through a chemical process or smoking. This removes the acid from the plant and renders it neutral and this causes the body to process the cannabinoids in a different manner.

Dioecious - a biological term that means having male and female organs in separate and distinct individuals; having separate sexes. Cannabis plants are dioecious

ECS - endogenous cannabinoid system

Endogenous cannabinoid system - the endocannabinoid system (ECS) is a group of endogenous cannabinoid receptors located in the mammalian brain and throughout the central and peripheral nervous systems, consisting of neuromodulatory lipids and their receptors. Known as "the body's own cannabinoid system," the ECS is involved in a variety of physiological processes including appetite, pain-sensation, mood, and memory, and in mediating the psychoactive effects of cannabis.

Entourage effect - refers to a concept and proposed mechanism by which compounds present in cannabis, which are largely non-psychoactive by themselves, modulate the overall psychoactive effects of the plant. Cannabidiol is believed to be the major modulatory component of cannabis, mitigating some of the negative, psychosis-like effects of THC, and is included in some medicinal formulations alongside THC. CBD co-administration also reduces the negative effects of THC on memory.

Hemp - a variety of the cannabis sativa plant species that is grown primarily for the industrial uses of its derived products. Hemp is a distinct cultivar of the cannabis plant that contains very little tetrahydrocannabinol (THC).

Homeostasis - the tendency of a system, especially the physiological system of higher animals, to maintain internal stability, owing to the coordinated response of its parts to any situation or stimulus that would tend to disturb its normal condition or function.

Microbiome - a community of microorganisms (such as bacteria, fungi, and viruses) that inhabit a particular environment and especially the collection of microorganisms living in or on the human body.

Neuroprotective - serving to protect nerve cells against damage, degeneration, or impairment of function. Various cannabinoids exhibit neuroprotective properties.

Phytocannabinoids - cannabinoids that occur naturally in the cannabis plant ("phyto"). Endo-cannabinoids occur naturally in ("endo") the human body.

Psychoactive - a chemical substance that changes brain function and results in alterations in perception, mood, consciousness or behavior.

Pyruvate - a very important biological molecule. It is involved in a number of biological processes and is essential in cellular respiration. (study.com)

Terpenes - a large and diverse class of organic compounds, produced by a variety of plants, including cannabis. Terpenes often have a strong odor and may protect the plants that produce them by deterring herbivores and by attracting predators and parasites of herbivores. The difference between terpenes and terpenoids is that terpenes are hydrocarbons, whereas terpenoids contain additional functional groups. Cannabis terpenes are numerous and are secreted by the same glands that produce cannabinoids. Research is revealing remarkable properties in terpenes and cannabis terpenes may play a critical roles in therapeutic effect.

Tetrahydrocannabinol (THC) - one of at least 113 cannabinoids identified in cannabis. THC is the principal psychoactive constituent of cannabis.

Tincture - typically an alcoholic extract of plant material or solution of such. Numerous cannabinoid tinctures are available including many CBD tinctures made from hemp.

Trichomes - small appendages on the cannabis flowers that store cannabinoids and terpenes.

Upregulate - the process of increasing the response to a stimulus; *specifically* an increase in a cellular response to a molecular stimulus due to increase in the number of receptors on the cell surface.

www.ingramcontent.com/pod-product-compliance
Lightning Source LLC
Chambersburg PA
CBHW060517280326
41933CB00014B/2999